World Health

Editor: Tracy Biram

Volume 348

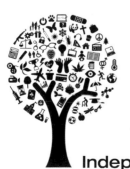

Independence Educational Publishers

First published by Independence Educational Publishers

The Studio, High Green

Great Shelford

Cambridge CB22 5EG

England

Y362.1

1776758

ISBN-13: 978 1 86168 804 0

Printed in Great Britain

Zenith Print Group

Contents

Introduction

WORLD HEALTH is Volume 348 in the **ISSUES** series. The aim of the series is to offer current, diverse information about important issues in our world, from a UK perspective.

ABOUT WORLD HEALTH

At least half of the world's population do not have full coverage of essential health services. Ebola, Zika virus, malaria and HIV are just some of the many diseases which affect the world's population.

This book explores the many health issues which affect different countries in the world. It also looks at the methods being used to try to prevent these diseases. From immunization programmes to drones fighting malaria, this book considers the ways in which we can track the outbreak of diseases and raise awareness as quickly as possible.

OUR SOURCES

Titles in the **ISSUES** series are designed to function as educational resource books, providing a balanced overview of a specific subject.

The information in our books is comprised of facts, articles and opinions from many different sources, including:

⇨ Newspaper reports and opinion pieces

⇨ Website factsheets

⇨ Magazine and journal articles

⇨ Statistics and surveys

⇨ Government reports

⇨ Literature from special interest groups.

A NOTE ON CRITICAL EVALUATION

Because the information reprinted here is from a number of different sources, readers should bear in mind the origin of the text and whether the source is likely to have a particular bias when presenting information (or when conducting their research). It is hoped that, as you read about the many aspects of the issues explored in this book, you will critically evaluate the information presented.

It is important that you decide whether you are being presented with facts or opinions. Does the writer give a biased or unbiased report? If an opinion is being expressed, do you agree with the writer? Is there potential bias to the 'facts' or statistics behind an article?

ASSIGNMENTS

In the back of this book, you will find a selection of assignments designed to help you engage with the articles you have been reading and to explore your own opinions. Some tasks will take longer than others and there is a mixture of design, writing and research-based activities that you can complete alone or in a group.

FURTHER RESEARCH

At the end of each article we have listed its source and a website that you can visit if you would like to conduct your own research. Please remember to critically evaluate any sources that you consult and consider whether the information you are viewing is accurate and unbiased.

Useful weblinks

www.avert.org

www.thebureauinvestigates.com

www.theconversation.com

www.theguardian.com

www.independent.co.uk

www.publishing.service.gov.uk

www.ucl.ac.uk

www.unicef.org

www.worldwatch.org

www.who.int

Progress towards the SDGs: A selection of data from *World Health Statistics 2018*

SDG3: Ensure healthy lives and promote well-being for all ages

Target 3.1: By 2030, reduce the global maternal mortality ratio to less than 70 per 100,000 live births

⇨ 303,000 women died due to complications of pregnancy or childbirth in 2015. Almost all of these deaths occurred in low- and middle-income countries (99%). Reducing maternal mortality crucially depends upon ensuring that women have access to quality care before, during and after childbirth.

⇨ Available data since 2007 shows that less than half of all births in several low- and middle-income countries were assisted by skilled health personnel. Globally it is estimated that over 40% of all pregnant women were not receiving early antenatal care in 2013.

Target 3.2: By 2030, end preventable deaths of newborns and children under five years of age, with all countries aiming to reduce neonatal mortality to at least as low as 12 per 1,000 live births and under-five mortality to at least as low as 25 per 1,000 live births

⇨ Under-five mortality rates continued to improve in 2016 dropping to 41 per 1,000 live births down from 93 per 1,000 live births in 1990. Nevertheless, every day in 2016, 15,000 children died before reaching their fifth birthday. Neonatal mortality has fallen from 37 per 1,000 live births in 1990 to 19 per 1,000 live births in 2016.

⇨ With more young children now surviving, improving the survival of older children (aged five to 14 years) is an increasing area of focus. About one million such children died in 2016, mainly from preventable causes.

Target 3.3: By 2030, end the epidemics of AIDS, tuberculosis, malaria and neglected tropical diseases and combat hepatitis, water-borne diseases and other communicable diseases

⇨ In 2016, an estimated one million people died of HIV-related illnesses. The global scale-up of antiretroviral therapy (ART) has been the main driver of the 48% decline in HIV-related deaths from a peak of 1.9 million in 2005. However, ART only reached 53% of people living with HIV at the end of 2016.

⇨ After unprecedented global gains in malaria control, progress has stalled. Globally, an estimated 216 million cases of malaria occurred in 2016, compared with 237 million cases in 2010 and 210 million cases in 2013. The main challenge that countries face in tackling malaria is a lack of sustainable and predictable funding.

Target 3.4: By 2030, reduce by one-third premature mortality from noncommunicable diseases through prevention and treatment and promote mental health and well-being

⇨ The probability of dying from diabetes, cancer, cardiovascular disease and chronic lung disease between ages 30 and 70 dropped to 18% in 2016, down from 22% in 2000. Adults in low- and lower-middle-income countries faced the highest risks – almost double the rate for adults in high-income countries. The total number of deaths from noncommunicable diseases is increasing due to population growth and ageing.

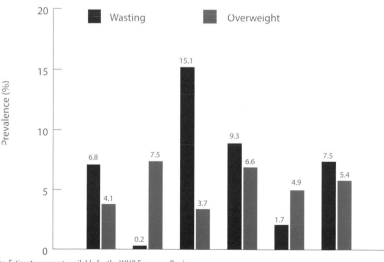

Fig. 1 Prevalence of wasting and overweight among children under five years old, by WHO regions and globally, 2017

Note: Estimates are not available for the WHO European Region due to low coverage of surveillance data

Source: World Health Organization

⇨ Almost 800,000 deaths by suicide occurred in 2016, with the highest rate in the European Region (15.4 per 100,000 population).

Target 3.5: Strengthen prevention and treatment of substance abuse, including narcotic drug abuse and harmful use of alcohol

⇨ The global level of alcohol consumption in 2016 has remained stable since 2010 at 6.4 litres of pure alcohol per person aged 15 years or older.

Target 3.6: By 2020, halve the number of global deaths and injuries from road traffic accidents

⇨ Deaths from road traffic injuries have increased since 2,000, reaching 1.25 million in 2013.

⇨ The death rate due to road traffic injuries was 2.6 times higher in low-income countries (24.1 deaths per 100,000 population) than in high-income countries (9.2 deaths per 100,000 population), despite lower rates of vehicle ownership in low-income countries.

Target 3.7: By 2030, ensure universal access to sexual and reproductive health care services, including for family planning, information and education, and the integration of reproductive health into national strategies and programmes

⇨ An estimated 208 million women of reproductive age who are married or in-union worldwide are still not having their family planning needs met with a modern contraceptive method. This represents 23% of all women of reproductive age who are married or in-union and wish to limit or space pregnancies.

⇨ There are an estimated 12.8 million births among adolescent girls aged 15–19 years every year. Early childbearing can increase risks for newborns as well as for young mothers.

Target 3.8: Achieve universal health coverage, including financial risk protection, access to quality essential health-care services and access to safe, effective, quality and affordable essential medicines and vaccines for all

⇨ At least half of the world's population do not have full coverage of essential health services.

⇨ In 2010, an estimated 808 million people – 11.7% of the world's population – spent at least 10% of their household budget paying out of their own pocket for health services. An estimated 97 million people were impoverished by out-of-pocket health care spending in 2010.

Target 3.9: By 2030, substantially reduce the number of deaths and illnesses from hazardous chemicals and air, water and soil pollution and contamination

⇨ In 2016, outdoor air pollution in both cities and rural areas caused an estimated 4.2 million deaths worldwide.

⇨ In the same year, indoor and outdoor air pollution caused an estimated seven million deaths, or one in eight deaths globally.

⇨ Unsafe water, sanitation and lack of hygiene were responsible for an estimated 870,000 deaths in 2016.

Target 3.a: Strengthen the implementation of the World Health Organization Framework Convention on Tobacco Control (WHO FCTC) in all countries, as appropriate

⇨ In 2016, more than 1.1 billion people smoked tobacco with 34% of all males 15 years and over against 6% of all females in this age group smoking.

⇨ During the period 2015–2016, over half (98) of WHO Member States strengthened their implementation of WHO FCTC through various measures, such as introducing or strengthening legislation requiring health warnings to appear on tobacco product packaging.

Target 3.b: Support the research and development of vaccines and medicines for the communicable and noncommunicable diseases that primarily affect developing countries, provide access to affordable medicines and vaccines, in accordance with the Doha Declaration on the TRIPS Agreement and Public Health, which affirms the right of developing countries to use to the full the provisions in the Agreement on Trade-Related Aspects of Intellectual Property Rights regarding flexibilities to protect public health, and, in particular, provide access to medicines for all

⇨ In 2016, one in ten children worldwide did not receive even the first dose of diphtheriatetanus-pertussis (DTP1) vaccine and coverage with the recommended three doses of the vaccine was 86%, a level which has essentially remained unchanged since 2010.

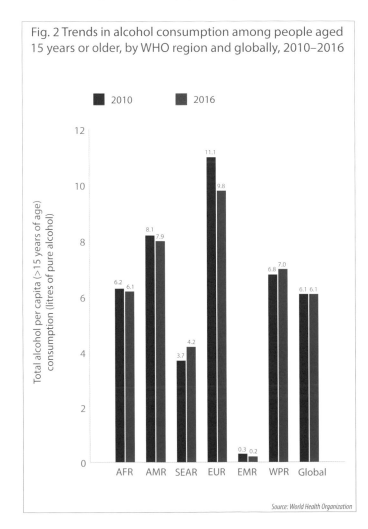

Fig. 2 Trends in alcohol consumption among people aged 15 years or older, by WHO region and globally, 2010–2016

■ 2010 ■ 2016

Total alcohol per capita (>15 years of age) consumption (litres of pure alcohol)

AFR: 6.2 / 6.1
AMR: 8.1 / 7.9
SEAR: 3.7 / 4.2
EUR: 11.1 / 9.8
EMR: 0.3 / 0.2
WPR: 6.8 / 7.0
Global: 6.1 / 6.1

Source: World Health Organization

Target 3.c: Substantially increase health financing and the recruitment, development, training and retention of the health workforce in developing countries, especially in least-developed countries and small-island developing States

⇨ In the period 2007–2016, 76 countries reported having less than one physician per 1,000 population.

⇨ In the same period, 87 countries reported having fewer than three nursing and midwifery personnel per 1,000 population.

Target 3.d: Strengthen the capacity of all countries, in particular developing countries, for early warning, risk reduction and management of national and global health risks

⇨ In 2017, 167 States Parties (85% of all States Parties) responded to the self-assessment questionnaire that is used to assess the implementation status of 13 core capacities. The average core capacity score of all reporting countries was 72%.

Selected health-related targets outside SDG3

Target 2.2: By 2030, end all forms of malnutrition, including achieving, by 2025, the internationally agreed targets on stunting and wasting in children under five years of age, and address the nutritional needs of adolescent girls, pregnant and lactating women and older persons

⇨ In 2017, 151 million children under five (22%) were stunted (too short for their age), with three-quarters of these children living in the South-East Asia Region or African Region.

⇨ 51 million children under the age of five (7.5%) were wasted (too light for their height) while 38 million children in this age group (5.6%) were overweight (too heavy for their height). Wasting and overweight may co-exist in a population at levels considered medium to high – the so-called 'double burden of malnutrition' – as observed in the Eastern Mediterranean Region.

Target 6.1: By 2030, achieve universal and equitable access to safe and affordable drinking-water for all

⇨ Safely managed drinking-water services – that is, located on premises, available when needed and free from contamination – were enjoyed by only 71% of the global population (5.2 billion people) in 2015.

Target 6.2: By 2030, achieve access to adequate and equitable sanitation and hygiene for all and end open defecation, paying special attention to the needs of women and girls and those in vulnerable situations

⇨ Safely managed sanitation services – with excreta safely disposed of *in situ* or treated off site – were available to only 39% of the global population (2.9 billion people) in 2015.

Target 7.1: By 2030, ensure universal access to affordable, reliable and modern energy services

⇨ Access to clean fuels and technologies for cooking has gradually improved. In 2016, 59% of the world's population were reliant primarily on clean fuels.

⇨ Population growth continues to outpace the transition to clean fuels and technologies, leaving three billion people still cooking with polluting fuel and stove combinations.

Target 11.6: By 2030, reduce the adverse per capita environmental impact of cities, including by paying special attention to air quality and municipal and other waste management

⇨ More than half of the urban population was exposed to outdoor air pollution levels at least 2.5 times above the safety standard set by WHO.

⇨ It is estimated that nine out of ten people worldwide breathe polluted air.

Target 13.1: Strengthen resilience and adaptive capacity to climate-related hazards and natural disasters in all countries

⇨ Over the period 2012–2016, on average there were 11,000 deaths globally each year due to natural disasters.

Target 16.1: Significantly reduce all forms of violence and related death rates everywhere

⇨ In 2016, an estimated 180,000 people were killed in wars and conflicts. This does not include deaths due to the indirect effects of war and conflict such as the spread of diseases, poor nutrition and collapse of health services. The global death rate due to conflicts in the past five years (2012–2016), at 2.5 deaths per 100,000 population, was more than double the average rate in the preceding five-year period (2007–2011).

⇨ There were an estimated 477,000 murders, with four-fifths of all homicide victims being male. Men in the Region of the Americas were the most affected (31.8 per 100,000 population).

Target 17.19: By 2030, build on existing initiatives to develop measurements of progress on sustainable development that complement gross domestic product, and support statistical capacity-building in developing countries

⇨ In 2016, 49% of deaths were registered with a cause of death, ranging from 6% of deaths in the African region to 98% in the European region.

2018

www.who.int

Nutrition
In the WHO African region

World Health Assembly commitments by WHO Member States:

2012
Countries agreed to work towards six global nutrition targets to be achieved by 2025

2015
Adopted a resolution to report biennially—beginning in 2018—on progress towards achievement of the targets

Objectives of the report

Profile countries' status in relation to the six global targets they committed to achieve by 2025

Explore sources of data to be used for progress monitoring and reporting at regional and global forums

Trigger reflection by governments and development partners on the investments needed to improve data collection and utilisation

What the report found

Periodic surveys are the primary source of data for nutrition monitoring ☑

Most countries' 'current' nutrition status is based on data more than five years old ☑

Malnutrition persists in the Region, for example:
• majority of countries have above 30% stunting prevalence, the number of stunted under-fives is increasing ☑
• only 17 countries have 'acceptable' levels of wasting (below 5%)
• childhood overweight is increasing in prevalence and the number of children affected ☑

Nutrition data are collected in primary health care visits but their utilisation to inform programme planning and interventions or surveillance and monitoring is extremely limited ☑

? The Big Questions

If we do not know where we are today, how can we plan for where to be in 2025? **1**

How will African countries report on their progress towards 2025 at the World Health Assembly and other accountability forums? **2**

Are governments and their partners willing to invest in nutrition monitoring? **3**

Recommended actions:

The Decade of Action on Nutrition is an opportunity for countries to make specific and measurable commitments to nutrition and track these alongside progress on the targets for 2025 (an interactive tracking tool for the targets is available at http://www.who.int/nutrition/trackingtool/en/)

Countries should invest in the use of routine nutrition data from primary health facilities to inform responsive nutrition programming, surveillance and monitoring

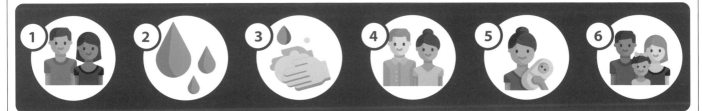

World Health Organization releases new global air pollution data

Nine out of ten people worldwide breathe polluted air, but more countries are taking action.

By CCAC secretariat, 2 May 2018

Air pollution levels remain dangerously high in many parts of the world. New data from the World Health Organization (WHO) released today, shows that nine out of ten people breathe air containing high levels of pollutants. Updated estimations reveal an alarming death toll of 7 million people every year caused by ambient (outdoor) and household air pollution.

'Air pollution threatens us all, but the poorest and most marginalized people bear the brunt of the burden,' says Dr Tedros Adhanom Ghebreyesus, Director-General of WHO. 'It is unacceptable that over three billion people – most of them women and children – are still breathing deadly smoke every day from using polluting stoves and fuels in their homes. If we don't take urgent action on air pollution, we will never come close to achieving sustainable development.'

> **'It is unacceptable that over three billion people – most of them women and children – are still breathing deadly smoke every day from using polluting stoves and fuels in their homes. If we don't take urgent action on air pollution, we will never come close to achieving sustainable development.'**
>
> **Dr Tedros Adhanom Ghebreyesus**
> **Director-General of WHO**

Seven million deaths every year

WHO estimates that around seven million people die every year from exposure to fine particles in polluted air that penetrate deep into the lungs and cardiovascular system, causing diseases including stroke, heart disease, lung cancer, chronic obstructive pulmonary diseases and respiratory infections, including pneumonia.

Ambient air pollution alone caused some 4.2 million deaths in 2016, while household air pollution from cooking with polluting fuels and technologies caused an estimated 3.8 million deaths in the same period.

More than 90% of air pollution-related deaths occur in low- and middle-income countries, mainly in Asia and Africa, followed by low- and middle-income countries of the Eastern Mediterranean region, Europe and the Americas.

Around three billion people – more than 40% of the world's population – still do not have access to clean cooking fuels and technologies in their homes, the main source of household air pollution. WHO has been monitoring household air pollution for more than a decade and, while the rate of access to clean fuels and technologies is increasing everywhere, improvements are not even keeping pace with population growth in many parts of the world, particularly in sub-Saharan Africa.

WHO recognises that air pollution is a critical risk factor for noncommunicable diseases (NCDs), causing an estimated one-quarter (24%) of all adult deaths from heart disease, 25% from stroke, 43% from chronic obstructive pulmonary disease and 29% from lung cancer.

More countries taking action

More than 4,300 cities in 108 countries are now included in WHO's ambient air quality database, making this the world's most comprehensive database on ambient air pollution. Since 2016, more than 1,000 additional cities have been added to WHO's database which shows that more countries are measuring and taking action to reduce air pollution than ever before.

The database collects annual mean concentrations of fine particulate matter (PM10 and PM2.5). PM2.5 includes pollutants, such as sulfate, nitrates and black carbon, which pose the greatest risks to human health. WHO air quality recommendations call for countries to reduce their air pollution to annual mean values of 20 μg/m^3 (for PM10) and 10 μg/m^3 (for PM25).

'Many of the world's megacities exceed WHO's guideline levels for air quality by more than five times, representing a major risk to people's health,' says Dr Maria Neira, Director of the Department of Public Health, Social and Environmental Determinants of Health, at WHO. 'We are seeing an acceleration of political interest in this global public health challenge. The increase in cities recording air pollution data reflects a commitment to air quality assessment and monitoring. Most of this increase has occurred in high-income countries, but we hope to see a similar scale-up of monitoring efforts worldwide.'

While the latest data show ambient air pollution levels are still dangerously high in most parts of the world, they also show some positive progress. Countries are taking measures to tackle and reduce air pollution from particulate matter. For example, in just two years, India's Pradhan Mantri Ujjwala Yojana Scheme has provided some 37 million women living below the poverty line with free LPG connections to support them to switch to clean household energy use. Mexico City has committed to cleaner vehicle standards, including a move to soot-free buses and a ban on private diesel cars by 2025.

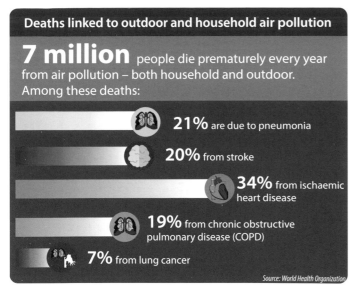

Deaths linked to outdoor and household air pollution

7 million people die prematurely every year from air pollution – both household and outdoor. Among these deaths:

- **21%** are due to pneumonia
- **20%** from stroke
- **34%** from ischaemic heart disease
- **19%** from chronic obstructive pulmonary disease (COPD)
- **7%** from lung cancer

Source: World Health Organization

Major sources of air pollution from particulate matter include the inefficient use of energy by households, industry, the agriculture and transport sectors, and coal-fired power plants. In some regions, sand and desert dust, waste burning and deforestation are additional sources of air pollution. Air quality can also be influenced by natural elements such as geographic, meteorological and seasonal factors.

Air pollution does not recognise borders. Improving air quality demands sustained and coordinated government action at all levels. Countries need to work together on solutions for sustainable transport, more efficient and renewable energy production and use, and waste management. WHO works with many sectors including transport and energy, urban planning and rural development to support countries to tackle this problem.

Key findings:

⇨ WHO estimates that around 90% of people worldwide breathe polluted air. Over the past six years, ambient air pollution levels have remained high and approximately stable, with declining concentrations in some part of Europe and in the Americas.

⇨ The highest ambient air pollution levels are in the Eastern Mediterranean Region and in South-East Asia,

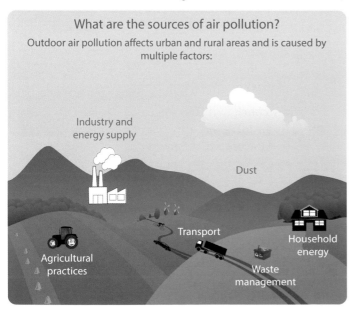

What are the sources of air pollution?

Outdoor air pollution affects urban and rural areas and is caused by multiple factors:

Industry and energy supply

Dust

Transport

Household energy

Agricultural practices

Waste management

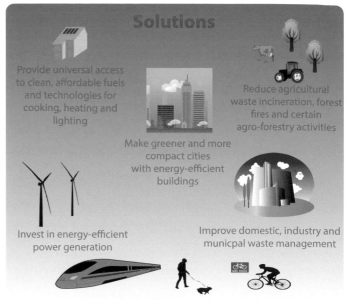

Solutions

Provide universal access to clean, affordable fuels and technologies for cooking, heating and lighting

Reduce agricultural waste incineration, forest fires and certain agro-forestry activities

Make greener and more compact cities with energy-efficient buildings

Invest in energy-efficient power generation

Improve domestic, industry and municpal waste management

Build safe and affordable public transport systems and pedestrian and cycle-friendly networks

Source: World Health Organization

with annual mean levels often exceeding more than five times WHO limits, followed by low- and middle-income cities in Africa and the Western Pacific.

⇨ Africa and some of the Western Pacific have a serious lack of air pollution data. For Africa, the database now contains PM measurements for more than twice as many cities as previous versions, however data was identified for only eight of 47 countries in the region.

⇨ Europe has the highest number of places reporting data.

⇨ In general, ambient air pollution levels are lowest in high-income countries, particularly in Europe, the Americas and the Western Pacific. In cities of high-income countries in Europe, air pollution has been shown to lower average life expectancy by anywhere between two and 24 months, depending on pollution levels.

'Political leaders at all levels of government, including city mayors, are now starting to pay attention and take action,' adds Dr Tedros. 'The good news is that we are seeing more and more governments increasing commitments to monitor and reduce air pollution as well as more global action from the health sector and other sectors like transport, housing and energy.'

WHO will convene the first Global Conference on Air Pollution and Health (30 October–1 November 2018) to bring governments and partners together in a global effort to improve air quality and combat climate change.

2 May 2018

www.who.int

Sleeping more than eight hours per night could increase risk of early death, finds study

Indulging in extra sleep could do more harm than good.

By Sarah Young

Sleeping for more than eight hours a night could lead to an early death, new research suggests.

A global study led by Keele University has found that people who regularly make time for more sleep could end up with a 'serious sleep disorder' that disrupts their breathing and causes an increased risk of heart disease.

As a result, the researchers, who looked at data from 74 studies, said that excessive sleep could be a 'marker' of poor health.

Published in the *Journal of the American Heart Association*, the study examined the link between self-reported sleep, cardiovascular disease and mortality in more than three million participants from 1970 to 2017.

The scientists found that a sleep duration of ten hours is linked with 30 per cent increased risks of early death compared to sleeping for seven hours.

The study also revealed a 56 per cent increased risk of stroke mortality and a 49 per cent increased risk of cardiovascular mortality for those who slept for more than eight hours.

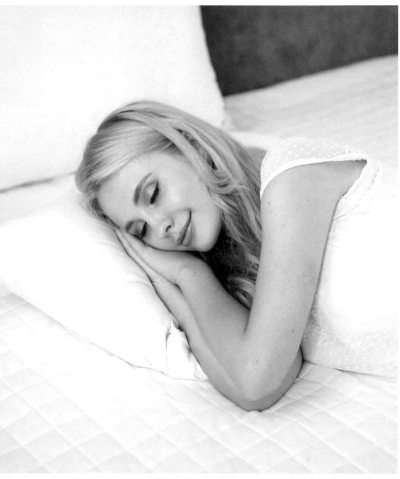

Lead researcher Dr Chun Shing Kwok, who works at Keele University's Institute for Science and Technology in Medicine, explains: 'Our study has an important public health impact in that it shows that excessive sleep is a marker of elevated cardiovascular risk.

'Our findings have important implications as clinicians should have greater consideration for exploring sleep duration and quality during consultations.

'If excessive sleep patterns are found, particularly prolonged durations of eight hours or more, then clinicians should consider screening for adverse cardiovascular risk factors and obstructive sleep apnoea, which is a serious sleep disorder that occurs when a person's breathing is interrupted during sleep.'

The study, which also found that poor sleep quality was associated with a 44 per cent increase in coronary heart disease, is one of many that highlight the impact sleep can have on a person's physical health.

Last month, the University of Sydney revealed that oxygen deprivation caused by sleep apnoea could cause your brain to shrink in the regions which play an important role in memory and which are also affected by dementia.

Similarly, a recent study by the University of Glasgow found that an insufficient amount of sleep could also be detrimental to your mental health.

The findings concluded that a disrupted circadian rhythm can lead to an increased possibility of developing mood disorders and lower levels of happiness.

7 August 2018

I nearly died from sepsis – and ignorance of this condition is killing millions

***An article from* The Conversation.**

THE CONVERSATION

By Michael J. Porter, Lecturer in Molecular Genetics, University of Central Lancashire

A visit to family in Glasgow for Christmas in 2015 nearly had a tragic ending for me. Two days earlier I had been repairing the lock on my garden gate, when I scratched my hand on a nail. By the time I arrived in Glasgow I was feeling unwell. 24 hours later I was in University Hospital Hairmyres in a coma. I had developed sepsis. My family were told that I had almost no chance of surviving the night.

I woke from my coma three months later and spent another year getting back to full health. I'm one of the lucky ones. Sepsis affects more than 30 million people a year worldwide and kills an estimated 6 million people, of whom nearly two million children. Of those who do survive, 40% will have post-sepsis syndrome, which leaves them with lasting physical and mental symptoms.

Sepsis starts with a viral or bacterial infection, usually of the lungs, abdomen or urinary tract, but it can also begin in a whole host of other ways, including a scratch (as happened in my case) or a bite. It's not the bug that causes the potentially life-threatening condition, however, it's the body's response to the infection. A complex cascade of events is triggered to fight an infection – in sepsis, this process becomes uncontrolled, rapidly accelerating and resulting in the failure of vital organs in the body, including the kidneys, heart and lungs.

Like a match being lit, a tiny spark at one end of the match head spreads out rapidly, the flame grows quickly and the match is destroyed by the flame, unless it's blown out in time. The 'flame' of sepsis in a body moves very quickly, and if my brother had not spotted those critical signs in time, or my treatment in the hospital had been delayed by even an hour, I would have died.

Sepsis symptoms can include pale and mottled skin, severe breathlessness, severe shivering or severe muscle pain, not urinating all day, nausea or vomiting. If you or someone you know has one or more of these symptoms, you should call the emergency services immediately and ask: 'Could it be sepsis?'

Anyone can get sepsis, although research suggests that people with a vitamin D deficiency have a higher risk of contracting sepsis than most. Vitamin D deficiency has also been linked to an increased risk of getting an infection, which may then go on to cause sepsis.

Promising avenues

Unfortunately, while it may be possible to treat the original infection with antibiotics, there is no specific cure for sepsis – only the symptoms can be treated. New research,

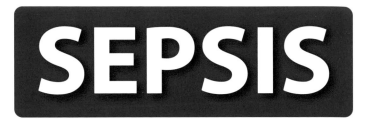

however, shows that metformin, a drug used to treat type 2 diabetes, can reduce the impact of sepsis by limiting the body's immune reaction and protecting it from damage by free radicals (oxygen-rich molecules that can damage cells).

Other promising research suggests that gene therapy may prove important in tackling sepsis, by targeting a protein produced in the body called NF-kB, which malfunctions during sepsis. If successful, these and other treatments in development have the potential to save lives and reduce the long-term impact of the disease on survivors.

The latest research seems promising, but the greatest defence we have against sepsis is awareness of the condition in medical professionals and the public. But at the moment awareness is alarmingly low across the world.

Surveys suggest that only 40% of people in Australia have heard of sepsis and only one-third of this group are able to identify a single symptom. Figures are even lower in Brazil where only 14% of the public know what it is. And, although campaigning in the UK and Germany has created an awareness in over 60% of people, knowledge of the warning signs is still limited.

As you'd expect, awareness is higher among healthcare professionals – but there is a need for greater education within this group. A definite diagnosis is often difficult, and efforts are being made to establish clear guidance for healthcare workers across the world, including the roll-out of an internationally recognised protocol called Sepsis6.

With time, scientific research may provide new treatments – but in the short term, greater awareness of the condition among the public and medical professionals is likely to have the biggest effect on saving lives and minimising harm. So always ask: 'Could it be sepsis?'

4 July 2018

Experts fear more food poisoning if chickens not inspected

By Andrew Wasley

Millions of chickens could soon be sold across the EU without being individually inspected for contamination or signs of disease after being killed, in a move some experts believe will put consumers at increased risk of food poisoning bugs.

Under current rules, every poultry carcass is individually, visually checked after slaughter and before being released for public consumption. But new proposals being considered by the European Commission would see slaughter plants able to look at just a 'representative sample' if they have a history of complying with the standards set by official veterinarians.

EU officials argue that increased microbiological screening of poultry flocks, improved food chain information and 'risk based' interventions are now more effective in preventing contaminated or sick birds from reaching consumers than post-mortem inspections of individual birds.

But some meat inspection bodies and consumer groups say the individual examinations are a vital tool for detecting fecal contamination, which can contain harmful bacteria, and indications of disease. Campylobacter is Europe's biggest cause of food poisoning, with up to nine million cases estimated to occur annually, although most are not reported. Rates of the disease – which can prove fatal – are known to be rising, with high levels found in chicken meat.

Ron Spellman, deputy secretary general of the European Association of Food and Meat Inspectors (EWFC), said the EU proposals, if approved, would lead to an increase in the 'already unacceptable' volume of food poisoning cases. 'Poultry causes a high level of human food poisoning due to its contamination with campylobacter and to a lesser extent, salmonella bacteria. These organisms are carried in the intestines of the birds which, during processing in the slaughterhouse, are sometimes ruptured causing the spread of visible faecal material onto the carcasses.'

Professor Chris Elliott, a food safety expert who led the official inquiry into the horsemeat scandal, told the Bureau he was concerned the proposed measures 'will only serve to lessen the degree of scrutiny at poultry plants and will thus mean a higher risk of meat not fit for human consumption entering the food chain. The objective is clearly to reduce costs.'

But Professor Hugh Pennington, who investigated fatal e.coli outbreaks in the UK, disagreed however, and said that he had 'always been unconvinced that visual inspection in itself brings significant food safety benefits.' This will mean a higher risk of meat not fit for human consumption entering the food chain'

'The current inspection regime still leaves campylobacter contamination of poultry at very high levels, so what is it delivering? Big salmonella reductions were due to things like immunisation [on farms], not more inspection,' he said.

The proposals follow a highly disputed 2012 report from the European Food Safety Authority (EFSA) which proposed that 'post-mortem visual inspection could be replaced by setting targets for the main hazards on the carcass, and by verification of the food business operator's hygiene management, using Process Hygiene Criteria'.

The current proposals were drawn up by the EU's Standing Committee on Plants, Animals, Food and Feed, which suggests that a 'derogation' from individual inspections could be approved if meat plants 'have a system in place to the satisfaction of the official veterinarian that allows the detection and the separation of birds with abnormalities, contamination or defects'.

If serious problems for human or animal health are found during earlier ante-mortem inspections (when birds arrive at the abattoir) then all birds would still require checking, the documents state.

EU spokesperson Anca Paduraru told the Bureau: 'The main hazards in poultry are salmonella and campylobacter. These pathogens will never be detected through the inspection of carcasses, but by bacteriological analysis [sampling]. This is why additional official controls for these two pathogens are now required in the proposed revision of the meat inspection [rules] with a view to strengthen the safety of poultry meat.'

She said the proposals, which are understood to be voted on later this year following a consultation, were optional and that individual countries would be left to make a decision on whether to adopt them.

Asked if it could rule out adopting the new system the Food Standards Agency (FSA) said: 'The UK will continue to comply with EU food and feed legislation while it remains a member of the EU. If any rule changes are considered after we leave, we will apply our usual rigorous risk assessment to those changes and ensure public safety remains at the heart of everything we do.'

In 2015 the FSA undertook a trial involving eight poultry processing plants in which inspections of individual poultry carcasses were reduced in favour of other official controls.

Richard Griffiths, Chief Executive of the British Poultry Council, signalled his support for the proposals, describing them as 'a positive step towards a more risk-based approach to meat inspection.

12 October 2018

UK's children denied basic human right to clean air, says Unicef

Young people face a long-term 'health crisis' unless the Government acts to clean up pollution, says children's charity.

By Matthew Taylor

C hildren in the UK are being denied their basic human right to breathe clean air and facing a long-term 'health crisis' because of the toxic fumes they breathe on their way to and from school, according to leading children's charity Unicef.

The organisation, which campaigns on children's rights and well-being around the world, described the situation in the UK as 'horrific' and has announced it is to make protecting youngsters from air pollution its priority across the country in the months ahead.

'I have been amazed as the picture has emerged showing us just exactly what the impact of air pollution is on children in the UK,' said Alastair Harper from Unicef UK.

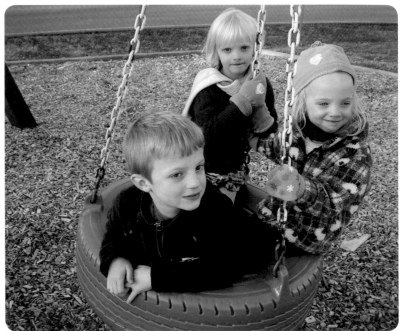

'Research is coming out all the time showing us how these toxic emissions can lead to lasting and devastating health impacts, impacts that will last their entire lives, from stunted lung growth to asthma to brain developments. It is horrific.'

Unicef's intervention follows a series of new studies which highlight the impact of the UK's air pollution crisis on children's health and will increase the pressure on government to intervene.

The charity, which is now working with schools across the country, as well as clean air groups, is calling on the Government to introduce a fully funded national action plan to protect children from the effects of toxic air.

Harper said: 'We want a national strategy specifically to protect children from harm, and a ring-fenced pot of funding to focus on the ways to reduce children's exposure to toxic air.

'We now know that exposure is most acute when they are travelling to and from school or nurseries and even inside the classrooms. Now there is no excuse not to take immediate and determined action.'

He said measures should include vehicle exclusion zones around schools, a network of clean air zones, improved walking and cycling infrastructure in towns and cities and more child-friendly urban areas.

Last year a *Guardian* investigation revealed hundreds of thousands of children are being exposed to illegal levels of damaging air pollution from diesel vehicles at more than 2,000 schools and nurseries across England and Wales.

Earlier this month it emerged that children were absorbing a disproportionate amount of air containing dangerous pollution on their way to and from school – and while in the classroom. One school was found to have several times over the World Health Organization pollution limit for the most damaging particulates inside several of its classrooms.

There is a growing campaign among some parents and schools to ban the school run and encourage walking and cycling, but Unicef said central government needs to step in to orchestrate a nationwide policy that protects young people's health.

'It has taken a while to understand the true nature of the problem but now we do know and we have to act.'

Harper said that unlike some other problems facing young people – including entrenched poverty and obesity – air pollution was relatively simple to address, if there was the political will.

'The fact is that it is so needless, we can fix this – other things are more intractable – but this is something we can resolve.'

The Government has been widely criticised for its lack of action on air pollution. It has lost three court cases and is one of five nations that have been referred to Europe's highest court for failing to tackle illegal levels of toxic air.

Harper said: 'All children have the right to breathe clean air, and toxic air not only violates children's right to breathe clean air it also impacts on their future and that is unacceptable.'

28 September 2018

Air pollution now threatening health worldwide

Humanity is losing the battle for clean air. Despite decades of efforts to combat it, air pollution is taking a growing toll on human health, the environment, and the economy, according to a new Worldwatch Institute study.

Once primarily an urban phenomenon in industrial countries, air pollution has spread worldwide. More than a billion people-one-fifth of all humanity live in communities that do not meet World Health Organization air quality standards.

In greater Athens, the number of deaths rises sixfold on heavily polluted days. Mexico City has been declared a hardship post for diplomats because of its unhealthy air. In Bombay, simply breathing is equivalent to smoking half a pack of cigarettes a day.

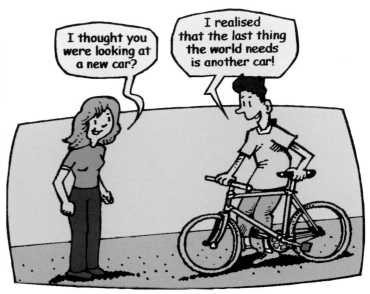

'The technological solutions tried to date have been inadequate, their gains often negated by growth,' according to Hilary F. French, a Researcher at the Washington, D.C.-based organisation and author of *Clearing the Air: A Global Agenda*. 'Restoring air quality depends on restructuring the energy, transportation, and industrial systems that generate the pollutants.'

In the US, air pollution causes as many as 50,000 deaths per year and costs as much as $40 billion a year in health care and lost productivity.

Around the world, Milan, Shenyang, Tehran, Seoul and Rio de Janeiro reported the worst levels of sulfur dioxide – a pollutant directly harmful to humans. Paris and Madrid also made the top ten in the list, produced by a UN monitoring network.

'Though concern for human health led to the world's first control laws, air pollution poses an equally grave threat to the environment,' said French.

'Lakes, streams and estuaries are dying because of acid rain, 35 percent of Europe's forests are showing signs of air pollution damage, and crop losses in the U.S. caused by harmful emissions are estimated to be 5–10 per cent of total production – more than $5 billion a year.'

Technological solutions – such as scrubbers, filters and catalytic converters – have long been the primary weapons to control emissions. Their use has become widespread in the industrialised world, but they are still virtually non-existent in most of Eastern Europe, the Soviet Union and the developing world.

'These technologies have helped, but they are increasingly being overwhelmed by industrialization and growth in car fleets. Policymakers nonetheless persist in combating specific pollutants with technological BandAids rather than addressing the problem at its roots.

'In the United States, for example, new clean air legislation currently before Congress mandates more pollution control technologies and may require the use of alternative fuels, but it pays scant attention to improving energy efficiency, decreasing reliance on cars, and reducing hazardous wastes.'

French advocates instead fundamental reforms in the regulation and design of polluting systems. For example, removing subsidies that keep fuel 3 prices artificially low and thus discourage energy efficiency would directly benefit air quality.

'China, for instance, has improved efficiency an average of 3.7 per cent a year since it began its economic reform programme in 1979. Similarly, adopting world market prices for energy could help clear the air in the Soviet Union.'

Incorporating the environmental costs of burning fossil fuels into energy planning could both encourage efficiency and the use of nonpolluting, renewable sources, according to French. An experiment under way in New York State forces power suppliers that burn fossil fuels to add one cent per kilowatt-hour to their contract bids to account for air pollution costs.

Taxing emissions can also be effective. Sweden is considering levies on sulfur dioxide, nitrogen oxides, and carbon dioxide from factories and power plants.

Taxes can also be used as an incentive to minimise pollution from automobiles. For instance, purchasers of low-emissions cars could receive a rebate funded by taxes on highly polluting ones. Sweden has such a system to encourage buying cars equipped with catalytic converters. Improved public transportation and urban planning designed to lessen dependence on autos, however, will be necessary to achieve lasting air quality gains.

'Freedom of information can be a crucial component in an air pollution strategy. In the United States, right-to-know legislation has been instrumental in spurring public outcry over toxic chemical emissions, leading to more responsible industrial behaviour,' French said.

Because air pollution respects no national boundaries, stepped up international cooperation is critical, according to French. Treaties have already been signed under the auspices of the European Economic Community and the UN Economic Commission for Europe to reduce the flow of pollutants across borders.

Some Western European countries are even finding it cheaper and more effective to fund control measures in upwind Eastern European countries than to take further steps at home.

West Germany, for example, is providing East Germany with $163 million in environmental aid to purchase advanced coal-burning technology for power plants and other pollution control measures.

In other cooperative ventures, the US-based Natural Resources Defense Council and Rocky Mountain Institute are advising the Soviet Government on energy efficiency.

'While the means are available to restore air quality, it will be a difficult task. In the West, powerful business interests will strongly resist measures that cost them money. In Eastern Europe, the Soviet Union, and the developing world, extreme economic problems coupled with shortages of currency mean that money for pollution prevention and control is scarce.

Around the world, however, the notion that "pollution is the price of progress" has become antiquated. Faced with ever mounting costs to human health and economic losses in agriculture and forestry, countries everywhere are discovering that pollution prevention is a sound investment.'

13 November 2018

Delhi smog: boxers forced to wear masks at world championships due to toxic air pollution

Level of deadly particulate matter at least eight times safe limit, India's pollution control board says.

By Harry Cockburn

Female boxers at the World Championships in Delhi have been forced to wear surgical masks, scarves or even t-shirts to cover their mouths during training as pollution levels have soared to several times above safe limits.

The boxers, who have gathered in the capital for the AIBA Women's World Boxing Championships, have said they have not been given protective gear, while the weather, with no wind to blow the smog away, has aggravated the problem in one of the world's most polluted cities.

On Tuesday 6 November, the level of deadly particulate matter PM 2.5, which lodges deep in the lungs, was at 407 micrograms per cubic metre, about eight times the safe limit, according to a reading by the country's pollution control board.

Readings reached 999 micrograms per cubic metre.

In Delhi, high levels of pollution are exacerbated every November and December by the seasonal burning of crop stubble in the neighbouring states of Punjab and Haryana.

Rubbish burning, dust from construction sites and huge diesel emissions from vehicles and industry have also contributed to the problem.

Though the championship is taking place in an indoor arena, teams are worried about the impact of the high level of pollution on athletes.

French coach Anthony Veniant said he had asked for the tournament to be moved out of Delhi but his request was turned down.

'We feel the air is no good. Some of the parents of these players are worried and we tell our players to restrict their time outside,' Veniant said.

Jay Kowli, secretary general of the Boxing Federation of India, said the air quality was being monitored but ruled out any change of location.

'Shifting the venue is impossible. Delhi has the best sports facilities in the country,' Mr Kowli said.

Competitors have been hard at training this week, despite concerns.

'My family is worried. We know it is not good for our body,' said 27-year old Bulgarian Stanimira Petrova, a gold-medallist in the bantamweight category in the championships in 2014.

British studies have previously recorded a seven per cent increase in mortality with each five micrograms per cubic metre increase in PM 2.5.

13 November 2018

New tuberculosis treatment could help tackle global epidemic

One-quarter of the world's population has latent tuberculosis – with 10.4 million new cases and 1.7 million deaths reported in 2016 alone.

By Sarah Boseley, Health Editor

A new, shorter and safer drug regime for latent tuberculosis could help curb the global epidemic by increasing the numbers successfully treated and reducing the pool of infection, researchers believe.

Two ground breaking studies, one in adults and the other in children, have trialled a less toxic drug than the one in current use worldwide for latent TB and cut the treatment time from nine months to four.

The research, pioneered by McGill University Health Centre in Canada, is set to change guidance around the world. One-quarter of the global population is thought to have latent TB infection, but because of the long course of drugs currently used, which can have toxic effects on the liver, many go untreated and some suffer harm.

People infected with latent TB may not become ill themselves, but if they then develop active TB they may transmit the infection to others. It is generally recognised that the chances of making real progress against the TB epidemic are slim unless the pool of latent infection can be reduced. There were an estimated 10.4 million new cases of active TB in 2016 and 1.7 million people died from the disease, according to the World Health Organization.

The standard treatment for latent TB at the moment is a lengthy course of isoniazid – for nine months in North America. The World Health Organization (WHO) recommends six months, largely for cost reasons. 'Whether you take it for four, six or nine months, it has significant side-effects, particularly on the liver,' said Dr Richard Menzies from McGill who led the new research. 'You can have liver failure.

'For preventive therapy you have quite healthy people who are carriers and encourage them to take medicines that can fry their liver for nine months. A lot of patients don't like it and even a lot of doctors don't like it.'

In the studies, adults and children with latent TB infection were given a different antibiotic called rifampin. The results, published in the *New England Journal of Medicine*, showed that four months of rifampin were as good as nine months of isoniazid. 'What we're showing is that you don't need isoniazid at all,' said Menzies.

'In my mind, safety is really number one when it comes to prevention.'

The adult trial involved more than 3,400 people taking isoniazid for nine months and the same number taking rifampin for four months, while enrolled more than 400 to

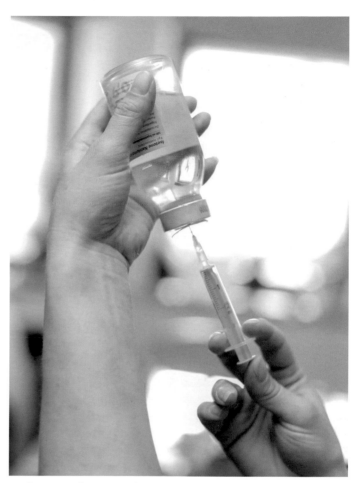

each arm. 'These are big trials,' said Menzies, who said he had been working to show there is a safer alternative for a decade, he said. 'Ten years ago I thought it was time to get rid of it [isoniazid],' he said.

In Quebec, which collects data on the treatment of patients in the same way as the NHS, there was on average one liver transplant a year as a result of latent TB treatment, he said. Developing countries struggle to treat active TB, let alone latent TB, but the middle-income countries like Brazil and India treat relatively few people with latent TB because of their fears of the side-effects of isoniazid.

Menzies, who has been involved in the writing of the US and Canadian guidelines on TB treatment, believes these and the WHO guidelines will now change. Australia and Japan are also interested in the findings, he said.

1 August 2018

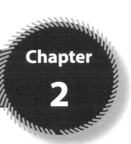

The 'greatest pandemic in history' was 100 years ago – but many of us still get the basic facts wrong

THE CONVERSATION

An article from **The Conversation.**

By Richard Gunderman, Chancellor's Professor of Medicine, Liberal Arts and Philanthropy, Indiana University

This year marks the 100th anniversary of the great influenza pandemic of 1918. Between 50 and 100 million people are thought to have died, representing as much as five per cent of the world's population. Half a billion people were infected.

Especially remarkable was the 1918 flu's predilection for taking the lives of otherwise healthy young adults, as opposed to children and the elderly, who usually suffer most. Some have called it the greatest pandemic in history.

The 1918 flu pandemic has been a regular subject of speculation over the last century. Historians and scientists have advanced numerous hypotheses regarding its origin, spread and consequences. As a result, many of us harbour misconceptions about it.

By correcting these ten myths, we can better understand what actually happened and learn how to prevent and mitigate such disasters in the future.

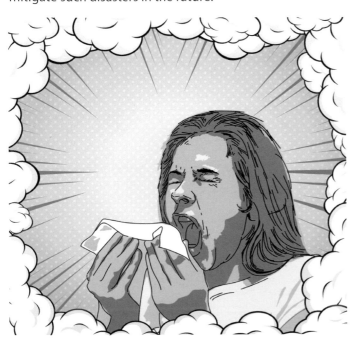

1. The pandemic originated in Spain

No one believes the so-called 'Spanish flu' originated in Spain.

The pandemic likely acquired this nickname because of World War I, which was in full swing at the time. The major countries involved in the war were keen to avoid encouraging their enemies, so reports of the extent of the flu were suppressed in Germany, Austria, France, the United Kingdom and the US. By contrast, neutral Spain had no need to keep the flu under wraps. That created the false impression that Spain was bearing the brunt of the disease.

In fact, the geographic origin of the flu is debated to this day, though hypotheses have suggested East Asia, Europe and even Kansas.

2. The pandemic was the work of a 'super-virus'

The 1918 flu spread rapidly, killing 25 million people in just the first six months. This led some to fear the end of mankind, and has long fuelled the supposition that the strain of influenza was particularly lethal.

However, more recent study suggests that the virus itself, though more lethal than other strains, was not fundamentally different from those that caused epidemics in other years.

Much of the high death rate can be attributed to crowding in military camps and urban environments, as well as poor nutrition and sanitation, which suffered during wartime. It's now thought that many of the deaths were due to the development of bacterial pneumonias in lungs weakened by influenza.

3. The first wave of the pandemic was most lethal

Actually, the initial wave of deaths from the pandemic in the first half of 1918 was relatively low.

It was in the second wave, from October through to December of that year, that the highest death rates were observed.

A third wave in spring of 1919 was more lethal than the first but less so than the second.

Scientists now believe that the marked increase in deaths in the second wave was caused by conditions that favoured the spread of a deadlier strain. People with mild cases stayed home, but those with severe cases were often crowded together in hospitals and camps, increasing transmission of a more lethal form of the virus.

4. The virus killed most people who were infected with it

In fact, the vast majority of the people who contracted the 1918 flu survived. National death rates among the infected generally did not exceed 20 per cent.

However, death rates varied among different groups. In the US, deaths were particularly high among Native American populations, perhaps due to lower rates of exposure to past strains of influenza. In some cases, entire Native communities were wiped out.

Of course, even a 20 per cent death rate vastly exceeds a typical flu, which kills less than one per cent of those infected.

5. Therapies of the day had little impact on the disease

No specific anti-viral therapies were available during the 1918 flu. That's still largely true today, where most medical care for the flu aims to support patients, rather than cure them.

One hypothesis suggests that many flu deaths could actually be attributed to aspirin poisoning. Medical authorities at the time recommended large doses of aspirin of up to 30 grams per day. Today, about four grams would be considered the maximum safe daily dose. Large doses of aspirin can lead to many of the pandemic's symptoms, including bleeding.

However, death rates seem to have been equally high in some places in the world where aspirin was not so readily available, so the debate continues.

6. The pandemic dominated the day's news

Public health officials, law enforcement officers and politicians had reasons to underplay the severity of the 1918 flu, which resulted in less coverage in the press. In addition to the fear that full disclosure might embolden enemies during wartime, they wanted to preserve public order and avoid panic.

However, officials did respond. At the height of the pandemic, quarantines were instituted in many cities. Some were forced to restrict essential services, including police and fire.

7. The pandemic changed the course of World War I

It's unlikely that the flu changed the outcome of World War I, because combatants on both sides of the battlefield were relatively equally affected.

However, there is little doubt that the war profoundly influenced the course of the pandemic. Concentrating millions of troops created ideal circumstances for the development of more aggressive strains of the virus and its spread around the globe.

8. Widespread immunisation ended the pandemic

Immunisation against the flu as we know it today was not practised in 1918, and thus played no role in ending the pandemic.

Exposure to prior strains of the flu may have offered some protection. For example, soldiers who had served in the military for years suffered lower rates of death than new recruits.

In addition, the rapidly mutating virus likely evolved over time into less lethal strains. This is predicted by models of natural selection. Because highly lethal strains kill their host rapidly, they cannot spread as easily as less lethal strains.

9. The genes of the virus have never been sequenced

In 2005, researchers announced that they had successfully determined the gene sequence of the 1918 influenza virus. The virus was recovered from the body of a flu victim buried in the permafrost of Alaska, as well as from samples of American soldiers who fell ill at the time.

Two years later, monkeys infected with the virus were found to exhibit the symptoms observed during the pandemic. Studies suggest that the monkeys died when their immune systems overreacted to the virus, a so-called 'cytokine storm.' Scientists now believe that a similar immune system overreaction contributed to high death rates among otherwise healthy young adults in 1918.

10. The 1918 pandemic offers few lessons for 2018

Severe influenza epidemics tend to occur every few decades. Experts believe that the next one is a question not of 'if' but 'when'.

While few living people can recall the great flu pandemic of 1918, we can continue to learn its lessons, which range from the commonsense value of handwashing and immunisations to the potential of anti-viral drugs. Today we know more about how to isolate and handle large numbers of ill and dying patients, and we can prescribe antibiotics, not available in 1918, to combat secondary bacterial infections. Perhaps the best hope lies in improving nutrition, sanitation and standards of living, which render patients better able to resist the infection.

For the foreseeable future, flu epidemics will remain an annual feature of the rhythm of human life. As a society, we can only hope that we have learned the great pandemic's lessons sufficiently well to quell another such worldwide catastrophe.

11 January 2018

Global HIV and AIDS statistics

2017 global HIV statistics

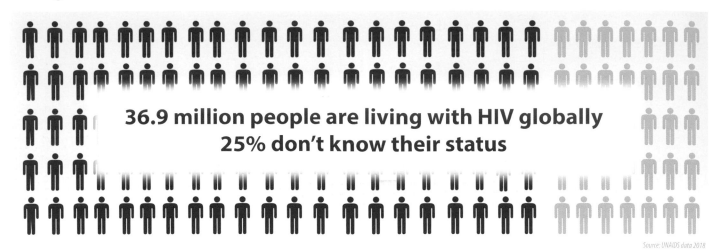

36.9 million people are living with HIV globally
25% don't know their status

Source: UNAIDS data 2018

HIV continues to be a major global public health issue. In 2017, an estimated 36.9 million people were living with HIV (including 1.8 million children) – with a global HIV prevalence of 0.8% among adults. Around 25% of these same people do not know that they have the virus.

Since the start of the epidemic, an estimated 77.3 million people have become infected with HIV and 35.4 million people have died of AIDS-related illnesses. In 2017, 940,000 people died of AIDS-related illnesses. This number has reduced by more than 51% (1.9 million) since the peak in 2004 and 1.4 million in 2010.

The vast majority of people living with HIV are located in low- and middle-income countries, with an estimated 66% living in sub-Saharan Africa. Among this group 19.6 million are living in East and Southern Africa which saw 800,000 new HIV infections in 2017.

Reaching the 90-90-90 targets

While there has been progress towards UNAIDS' 90-90-90 targets for prevention and treatment, this appears to be stalling and at current rates the targets will not be achieved by the 2020 deadline.

The first 90

In 2017, three out of four people living with HIV (75%) knew their status.

The second 90

Among people who knew their status, four out of five (79%) were accessing treatment.

The third 90

And among people accessing treatment, four out of five (81%) were virally suppressed. West and Central Africa, Eastern Europe and Central Asia are regions where urgent action is particularly important if we are to reach the targets.

New infections

There is renewed concern that the annual number of new infections among adults has remained static in recent years. In 2017, there were roughly 1.8 million new HIV infections – the same as in 2016.

Global new HIV infections have declined by just 18% in the past seven years, from 2.2 million in 2010 to 1.8 million in 2017. Although this is nearly half the number of new infections compared to the peak in 1996 (3.4 million), the decline is not quick enough to reach the target of fewer than 500,000 by 2020.

While new HIV infections among children globally have also declined, from 270,000 in 2010 to 180,000 in 2017 (35%), reports indicate that this is far less progress being made than previously thought and there is much more that needs to be done to improve knowledge of HIV and HIV testing among adolescents and young adults.

Young women are especially at risk, with around 7,000 new infections each week among young people aged 15–24 occurring among this group. In sub-Saharan Africa, three in four new infections are among girls aged 15–19 years and young women aged 15–24 years are twice as likely to be living with HIV than men.

More than one-third (35%) of women around the world have experienced physical and/or sexual violence at some time in their lives. In some regions, women who experience

Global progress towards the 90-90-90 targets 2017 (all ages)

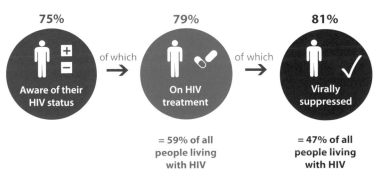

Source: UNAIDS data 2018

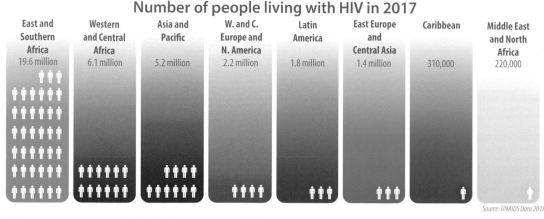

Number of people living with HIV in 2017

| East and Southern Africa 19.6 million | Western and Central Africa 6.1 million | Asia and Pacific 5.2 million | W. and C. Europe and N. America 2.2 million | Latin America 1.8 million | East Europe and Central Asia 1.4 million | Caribbean 310,000 | Middle East and North Africa 220,000 |

Source: UNAIDS Data 2018

violence are one and a half times more likely to become infected with HIV.

The reduction in new HIV infections has been strongest in the region most affected by HIV, East and Southern Africa, where new HIV infections have been reduced by 30% since 2010. However, new HIV infections are rising in around 50 countries. In Eastern Europe and Central Asia the annual number of new HIV infections has doubled, and new HIV infections have increased by more than a quarter in the Middle East and North Africa over the past 20 years.

Moreover, despite the progress made across the 69 countries which have witnessed a decline in new infections, progress in combating viral transmission is still not happening fast enough to meet global targets.

Treatment

Despite challenges, new global efforts have meant that the number of people receiving HIV treatment has increased dramatically in recent years, particularly in resource-poor countries.

In 2017, 59% of all people living with HIV were accessing treatment. Of those, 47% were virally suppressed.

In 2017, 21.7 million people living with HIV were receiving antiretroviral treatment (ART) – an increase of 2.3 million since 2016 and up from eight million in 2010. However, this

level of treatment scale up is still not enough for the world to meet its global target of 30 million people on treatment by 2020.

Significant progress has been made in the prevention of mother-to-child transmission of HIV (PMTCT). In 2017, 80% of all pregnant women living with HIV had access to treatment to prevent HIV transmission to their babies – this is up from 47% in 2010.

HIV and tuberculosis (TB)

Tuberculosis (TB) remains the leading cause of death among people living with HIV, accounting for around one in three AIDS-related deaths. In 2016, 10.4 million people developed TB; of those 1.2 million were living with HIV.

Funding

At the end of 2017, US$21.3 billion was available for the AIDS response in low- and middle-income countries. This was a slight increase from the US$19 billion in global funding available in 2016. Around 56% of the total resources for HIV in low- and middle-income countries in 2017 were from domestic sources.

UNAIDS estimates that US$26.2 billion will be required for the AIDS response in 2020.

8 October 2018

www.avert.org

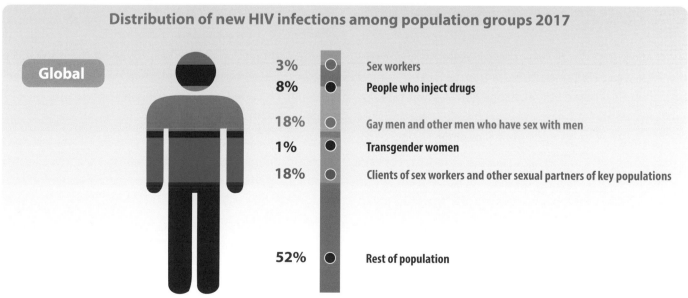

Distribution of new HIV infections among population groups 2017

Global

3%	Sex workers
8%	**People who inject drugs**
18%	Gay men and other men who have sex with men
1%	**Transgender women**
18%	Clients of sex workers and other sexual partners of key populations
52%	**Rest of population**

Source: UNAIDS special analysis, 2018

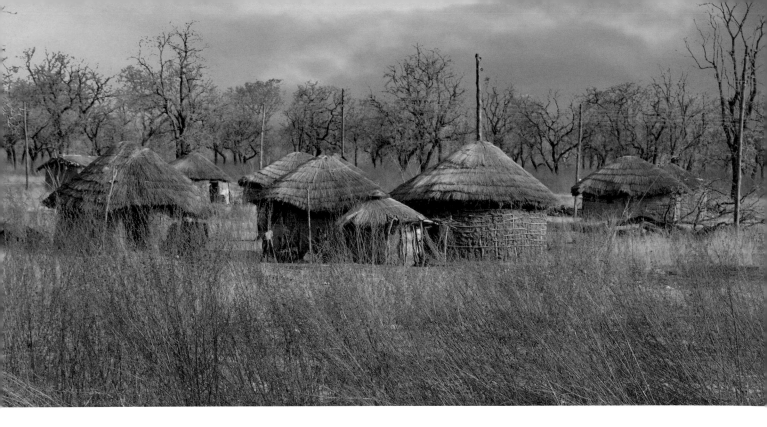

As Ebola has shown, the global health system is as strong as its weakest link

The West African Ebola outbreak started in a small village in Guinea. It shows the value of investing in grassroots healthcare.

By Ellen Johnson Sirleaf, former President of Liberia

In the city of Beni, in the north-east corner of the Democratic Republic of the Congo, an outbreak of Ebola is simmering. Fear of this lethal disease and all that goes with it – grief over lost loved ones, exhausted emergency response workers and ongoing insecurity – might once have felt distant, foreign, unknowable. But, tragically, these emotions are all too familiar.

Almost five years ago, a two-year-old boy from Meliandou – a tiny rural village in southern Guinea, bordering Liberia and Sierra Leone – fell sick with a strange illness. His symptoms were the stuff of nightmares: internal bleeding, black stools, vomiting and a high fever. Just two days later, he died.

At the time, no one in the village knew what the cause of death was; no one could anticipate the chain of consequences that was about to rip through the region and fuel a global panic.

From Meliandou, the disease slipped across Guinea's porous border and spread unabated through West Africa for four months, before it was correctly identified as Ebola. The world watched in horror as the largest Ebola outbreak in history engulfed my country and the rest of the region, infecting over 27,000 people in total and killing more than 11,000.

Ebola consumed every aspect of daily life. The economy faltered as international trade halted, schools were shut and hard-fought progress on child and maternal mortality was wiped out overnight. Beyond West Africa, isolated outbreaks around the world spread panic and reflected the darker consequences of how interconnected global health has become.

We learned that the world's health system is only as strong as its weakest link. Investing in primary healthcare is the best way to detect and stop local outbreaks before they become global pandemics.

Local healthcare services are a person's first and main point of contact with the health system – the place in their community where they can go to see a provider able to address the majority of their health needs. When this primary system is strong, patients develop trusted relationships with their healthcare providers, who can encourage them to seek the care they need, including in times of crisis. Primary healthcare providers are also best positioned to spot the early warning signs of outbreaks – and sound the alarm bell when needed.

In Liberia, we saw that communities with strong primary healthcare were better able to stem the spread of Ebola. We are now applying these lessons to more effectively protect the health of our people should another outbreak strike. We have prioritised investments in primary healthcare to ensure that citizens can secure essential health services free of charge and see primary healthcare providers in their own communities, even in the most remote parts of the country.

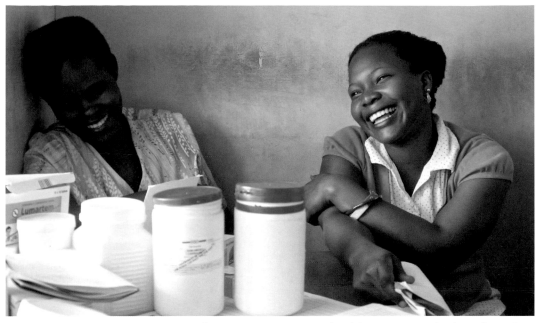

Liberia's national community health assistant programme was launched in July 2016 and will serve more than 4,000 remote communities in the hardest to reach areas of our country by 2021. Each community health assistant is critical to the health of their community, and is trained, paid and supervised to deliver common screening, treatment and preventive health services.

The 3,000 community health assistants deployed to date have identified more than 1,700 warning signs of outbreaks in the past year alone, and have been instrumental in addressing these before they spin out of control. They are critical links to keeping communities across remote Liberia healthy, ensuring that we are better prepared to weather the next storm.

But I know we do not have the complete blueprint to build stronger health systems on our own. Countries must learn from each other – and not just in times of crisis. I am closely watching the work of the primary healthcare performance initiative, which is partnering with country governments to measure the strengths and weaknesses of existing health systems. The initiative's new 'vital signs profiles', which are launching this week, are designed to help leaders pinpoint opportunities for maximum impact when investing in the systems that guard the health of our people.

West Africa still feels the lasting effects of Ebola, while our brothers and sisters in DRC are working urgently to bring an end to the current outbreak before it spirals out of control. Unless we learn the hard lessons, the global health system will remain like a house without a foundation. Ensuring that everyone, everywhere, has access to essential health services is our best shot at avoiding the all too familiar cycle of health emergencies. Now is the time to act with conviction.

25 October 2018

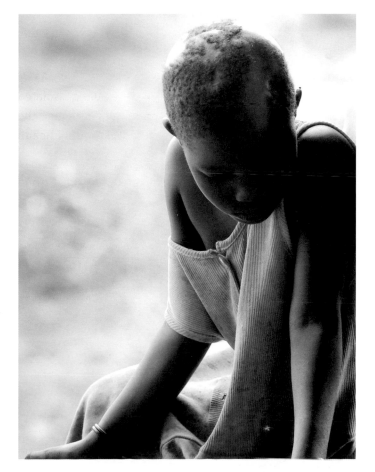

Zika virus

Key facts

⇨ Zika virus disease is caused by a virus transmitted primarily by *Aedes* mosquitoes, which bite during the day.

⇨ Symptoms are generally mild and include fever, rash, conjunctivitis, muscle and joint pain, malaise or headache. Symptoms typically last for 2–7 days. Most people with Zika virus infection do not develop symptoms.

⇨ Zika virus infection during pregnancy can cause infants to be born with microcephaly and other congenital malformations, known as congenital Zika syndrome. Infection with Zika virus is also associated with other complications of pregnancy including preterm birth and miscarriage.

⇨ An increased risk of neurologic complications is associated with Zika virus infection in adults and children, including Guillain-Barré syndrome, neuropathy and myelitis.

Zika virus is a mosquito-borne flavivirus that was first identified in Uganda in 1947 in monkeys. It was later identified in humans in 1952 in Uganda and the United Republic of Tanzania.

Outbreaks of Zika virus disease have been recorded in Africa, the Americas, Asia and the Pacific. From the 1960s to 1980s, rare sporadic cases of human infections were found across Africa and Asia, typically accompanied by mild illness.

The first recorded outbreak of Zika virus disease was reported from the Island of Yap (Federated States of Micronesia) in 2007. This was followed by a large outbreak of Zika virus infection in French Polynesia in 2013 and other countries and territories in the Pacific. In March 2015, Brazil reported a large outbreak of rash illness, soon identified as Zika virus infection, and in July 2015, found to be associated with Guillain-Barré syndrome.

In October 2015, Brazil reported an association between Zika virus infection and microcephaly. Outbreaks and evidence of transmission soon appeared throughout the Americas, Africa and other regions of the world. To date, a total of 86 countries and territories have reported evidence of mosquito-transmitted Zika infection.

Signs and symptoms

The incubation period (the time from exposure to symptoms) of Zika virus disease is estimated to be three to 14 days. The majority of people infected with Zika virus do not develop symptoms. Symptoms are generally mild including fever, rash, conjunctivitis, muscle and joint pain, malaise, and headache, and usually last for two to 7 days.

Complications of Zika virus disease

Zika virus infection during pregnancy is a cause of microcephaly and other congenital abnormalities in the developing fetus and newborn. Zika infection in pregnancy also results in pregnancy complications such as fetal loss, stillbirth and preterm birth.

Zika virus infection is also a trigger of Guillain-Barré syndrome, neuropathy and myelitis, particularly in adults and older children.

Research is ongoing to investigate the effects of Zika virus infection on pregnancy outcomes, strategies for prevention and control, and effects of infection on other neurological disorders in children and adults.

Transmission

Zika virus is primarily transmitted by the bite of an infected mosquito from the *Aedes* genus, mainly *Aedes aegypti*, in tropical and subtropical regions. *Aedes* mosquitoes usually bite during the day, peaking during early morning and late afternoon/evening. This is the same mosquito that transmits dengue, chikungunya and yellow fever.

Zika virus is also transmitted from mother to fetus during pregnancy, through sexual contact, transfusion of blood and blood products, and organ transplantation.

Diagnosis

Infection with Zika virus may be suspected based on symptoms of persons living in or visiting areas with Zika virus transmission and/or *Aedes* mosquito vectors. A diagnosis of Zika virus infection can only be confirmed by laboratory tests of blood or other body fluids, such as urine or semen.

Treatment

There is no treatment available for Zika virus infection or its associated diseases.

Symptoms of Zika virus infection are usually mild. People with symptoms such as fever, rash or arthralgia should get plenty of rest, drink fluids, and treat pain and fever with common medicines. If symptoms worsen, they should seek medical care and advice.

Pregnant women living in areas with Zika transmission or who develop symptoms of Zika virus infection should seek medical attention for laboratory testing and other clinical care.

Prevention

Mosquito bites

Protection against mosquito bites during the day and early evening is a key measure to prevent Zika virus infection. Special attention should be given to prevention of mosquito bites among pregnant women, women of reproductive age and young children.

Personal protection measures include wearing clothing (preferably light-coloured) that covers as much of the body as possible; using physical barriers such as window screens and closed doors and windows; and applying insect repellent to skin or clothing that contains DEET, IR3535 or icaridin according to the product label instructions.

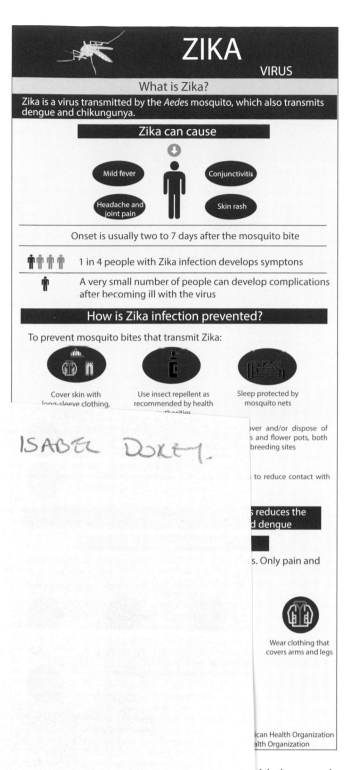

ZIKA
VIRUS

What is Zika?

Zika is a virus transmitted by the *Aedes* mosquito, which also transmits dengue and chikungunya.

Zika can cause

- Mild fever
- Conjunctivitis
- Headache and joint pain
- Skin rash

Onset is usually two to 7 days after the mosquito bite

1 in 4 people with Zika infection develops symptons

A very small number of people can develop complications after becoming ill with the virus

How is Zika infection prevented?

To prevent mosquito bites that transmit Zika:

- Cover skin with long-sleeve clothing,
- Use insect repellent as recommended by health authorities
- Sleep protected by mosquito nets

...ver and/or dispose of ...s and flower pots, both ...breeding sites

...to reduce contact with

...s reduces the ...d dengue

...s. Only pain and

Wear clothing that covers arms and legs

...ican Health Organization ...alth Organization

ISABEL DOLEY.

...uld sleep under ...r early evening.

Travellers and those living in affected areas should take the same basic precautions described above to protect themselves from mosquito bites.

Aedes mosquitoes breed in small collections of water around homes, schools and work sites. It is important to eliminate these mosquito breeding sites, including: covering water storage containers, removing standing water in flower pots, and cleaning up trash and used tyres. Community initiatives are essential to support local government and public health programmes to reduce mosquito breeding sites. Health authorities may also advise use of larvicides and insecticides to reduce mosquito populations and disease spread.

No vaccine is yet available for the prevention or treatment of Zika virus infection. Development of a Zika vaccine remains an active area of research.

Transmission in pregnancy

Zika virus can be transmitted from mother to fetus during pregnancy, resulting in microcephaly (smaller than normal head size) and other congenital malformations in the infant, collectively referred to as congenital Zika syndrome.

Microcephaly is caused by underlying abnormal brain development or loss of brain tissue. Child outcomes vary according to the extent of the brain damage.

Congenital Zika syndrome includes other malformations including limb contractures, high muscle tone, eye abnormalities and hearing loss. The risk of congenital malformations following infection in pregnancy remains unknown; an estimated 5–15% of infants born to women infected with Zika virus during pregnancy have evidence of Zika-related complications. Congenital malformations occur following both symptomatic and asymptomatic infection.

Sexual transmission

Zika virus can be transmitted through sexual intercourse. This is of concern due to an association between Zika virus infection and adverse pregnancy and fetal outcomes.

For regions with active transmission of Zika virus, all people with Zika virus infection and their sexual partners (particularly pregnant women) should receive information about the risks of sexual transmission of Zika virus.

WHO recommends that sexually active men and women be correctly counselled and offered a full range of contraceptive methods to be able to make an informed choice about whether and when to become pregnant in order to prevent possible adverse pregnancy and fetal outcomes.

Women who have had unprotected sex and do not wish to become pregnant due to concerns about Zika virus infection should have ready access to emergency contraceptive services and counselling. Pregnant women should pratise safer sex (including correct and consistent use of condoms) or abstain from sexual activity for at least the entire duration of pregnancy.

For regions with no active transmission of Zika virus, WHO recommends practising safer sex or abstinence for a period of six months for men and two months for women who are returning from areas of active Zika virus transmission to prevent infection of their sex partners. Sexual partners of pregnant women, living in or returning from areas where local transmission of Zika virus occurs, should practise safer sex or abstain from sexual activity throughout pregnancy.

20 July 2018

www.who.int

Disease detectives: keeping track of new and emerging infectious diseases

By Jennifer Lloyd, PHE epidemiologist

Ebola! Marburg! Zika virus! Black Death!

These are words you may have heard quite a lot these past few years. Almost every day, somewhere in the world, there are stories in the media about diseases which can kill us or rumours of a new 'eye-bleeding disease'. While these might be entertaining to read, they are very frustrating for us as Emerging Infections scientists, because they spread a lot of misinformation and fear.

While this is all very interesting, at this point you may be thinking to yourself, but why should I care? The media stories are just rumours. There has been nothing in the news lately about Ebola or Zika virus outbreaks. Those diseases are gone, aren't they?

Well, no. Most of these emerging infections are present in the animal or insect population for years before (and after) an outbreak occurs. They may even cause human cases that aren't detected. Because of this, in the past some outbreaks haven't been recognised until they were already established. That's where we come in.

Epidemic Intelligence

Here in the Emerging Infections and Zoonoses section, it's our job to detect these events as early and quickly as possible to raise awareness for clinicians, labs and across government. To do this, we conduct epidemic intelligence. This is a process of horizon scanning (a form of surveillance) that is used to identify and gather information about current outbreaks and incidents of new and emerging infectious diseases, occurring anywhere in the world.

This means that we spend half of each day combing nearly a hundred sources on the internet for rumours of diseases and 'unusual incidents' around the world. We look at everything – official reports from international organisations like the WHO and Ministries of Health, international and local media, and even Facebook and Twitter. We use these because the majority of the world's first news about infectious disease events now comes from unofficial sources, including newspapers, social media and other Internet resources.

Why rumours matter to us

One of the main things we look for are rumours; rumours from local or social media of undiagnosed diseases, unusual events, haemorrhagic fevers (serious viral infections characterised by sudden onset of fever and bleeding) and/or large numbers of deaths. When we find something, we record it in our database and then go to work searching other sources for more information.

Then we conduct a risk assessment to determine if further escalation is necessary. If the answer is yes, then the information is communicated within PHE and to appropriate people within the UK Government. We help them gain awareness of disease events around the world and provide expert advice on situations that might get out of hand.

So how does it work

Horizon scanning becomes even more important when working with an emerging infection, like Zika virus, as every day our knowledge of this previously little known virus grew. As at the start of the Ebola outbreak in West Africa in March 2014, our epidemic intelligence system picked up an outbreak of undiagnosed illness in Brazil before it was officially confirmed as Zika virus. We first detected media reports about an undiagnosed outbreak of fever/rash in Brazil in early 2015. Zika virus in Brazil was first confirmed in May 2015. Based on what we knew about other Aedes mosquito-borne diseases such as dengue and chikungunya, we were sure that this outbreak would quickly spread far and wide, but no-one anticipated the impact Zika would have on an unborn ch ild.

The truth is these diseases have been present in parts of the world for years. They are called emerging infections. Emerging infections are either newly recognised diseases or diseases that are increasing in a specific place, or among a specific population. They can be transmitted in many ways, including by insects, water, animals or from person-to-person. Most emerging infections are zoonotic, meaning they spread from animals to humans.

With the increased movement of people around the globe and increased urbanisation, the likelihood of coming into contact with new/emerging diseases has increased. This is because humans come into contact more readily with creatures that harbour these infections, whether they are mosquitoes, ticks or animals. And the more we come into contact with them, the more likely we are to become infected.

With a situation like Zika, new information is received and reviewed on a daily basis to ensure we provide the most relevant and accurate information to those concerned about the situation. This could mean posting the information on relevant gov.uk webpages (such as the Zika collection), sharing it with our colleagues at NaTHNaC who provide country specific travel guidance or distributing it elsewhere.

21 February 2018

www.gov.uk

Scientists use gene-editing to destroy mosquito population in lab

Technique could be used to control spread of malaria, researchers believe.

By Samuel Osborne

Scientists have successfully wiped out a population of mosquitoes in a laboratory using a type of genetic engineering.

The researchers managed to eliminate the population within 11 generations, suggesting in a paper published in the journal *Nature Biology* that the technique could be used to control the spread of malaria.

They used a type of gene editing known as gene drive, which spread a modification designed to block female reproduction.

'It will still be at least five to ten years before we consider testing any mosquitoes with gene drive in the wild, but now we have some encouraging proof that we're on the right path,' said Andrea Crisanti, a professor at Imperial College London who co-led the work.

The research marks the first time the technology has been able to completely suppress a population.

It is hoped that in the future, mosquitoes carrying a gene drive could be released to spread female infertility within local malaria-carrying mosquito populations in order to cause them to collapse.

Gene drive technologies alter DNA and drive self-sustaining genetic changes through multiple generations.

They do so by overriding normal biological processes.

However, they are also considered controversial since such genetically-engineered organisms could have an unknown and irreversible impact on the ecosystem once they are released into the wild.

The technique used in the study was designed to target the specific mosquito species *Anopheles gambiae*, which is responsible for malaria transmission in sub-Saharan Africa.

The World Health Organization has warned that global progress against malaria is stalling and could be reversed if momentum in the fight to wipe it out was lost.

The disease infected around 216 million people worldwide in 2016 and killed 445,000 of them. The vast majority of malaria deaths are in babies and young children in sub-Saharan Africa.

Males who carried this modified gene showed no changes, and neither did females with only one copy of it, he explained.

But females with two copies of the modified gene showed both male and female characteristics – they failed to bite and did not lay eggs.

The experiments found the gene drive transmitted the genetic modification nearly 100 per cent of the time, and after between seven and 11 generations the populations collapsed due to lack of offspring.

Mr Crisanti said the results showed that gene drive solutions can work, offering 'hope in the fight against a disease that has plagued mankind for centuries'.

He added, however, that 'there is still more work to be done, both in terms of testing the technology in larger lab-based studies and working with affected countries to assess the feasibility of such an intervention'.

But Mariann Bassey, a campaigner with the environmental group Friends of the Earth Africa, said the technique was risky.

'To solve the malaria crisis, we should focus on the least risky and most effective solutions, not experiment with ecosystems with little regard for the potentially new environmental and health consequences,' she said in a statement.

25 September 2018

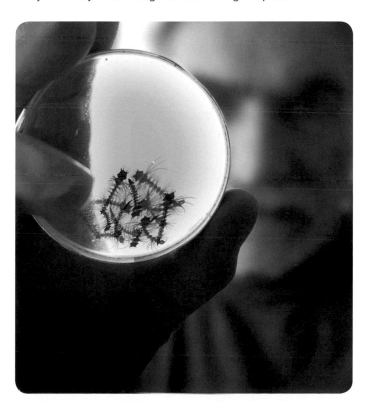

Malaria imported into the United Kingdom: 2017

This is an extract from the above article.

Introduction

Malaria is a serious and potentially life threatening febrile illness caused by infection with the protozoan parasite *Plasmodium*. It is transmitted to humans by the bite of the female *Anopheles* mosquito in tropical and subtropical regions of the world. There are five species of *Plasmodium* that infect humans: *P. falciparum* (responsible for the most severe form of malaria and the most deaths), *P. vivax*, *P. ovale*, *P. malariae* and *P. knowlesi*.

Malaria does not currently occur naturally in the UK but travel-associated cases are reported in those who have returned to the UK or arrived (either as a visitor or migrant to the UK) from malaria endemic areas.

General trend

In 2017, 1,792 cases of imported malaria were reported in the UK (1,708 in England, 50 in Scotland, 24 in Wales and 10 in Northern Ireland), 10.8% higher than reported in 2016 (N=1,618) and 15.0% above the mean number of 1,558 cases reported between 2008 and 2017.

In the last ten years (between 2008 and 2017), the total number of malaria cases reported in the UK each year has fluctuated around a mean of 1,558 (95% CI: 1,447–1,668); similar to the mean for the previous ten years (1,533, 95% CI: 1,440–1,627).

The great majority of the cases in 2017 were caused by *P. falciparum*, which is consistent with previous years, and although the total number of cases caused by *P. falciparum* increased compared to 2016, the proportion of the total number of cases remained stable. The proportion of cases caused by *P. vivax* and *P. ovale* also remained similar over the two years, with the proportion of cases caused by *P. vivax* decreasing slightly in 2017 (Table 1).

Table 1. Malaria cases in the UK by species: 2017 and 2016

Malaria parasite	Cases (% of total)	
	2017	**2016**
P. falciparum	1,452 (81.0%)	1.308 (80.8%)
P. vivax	164 (9.2%)	166 (10.3%)
P. ovale	108 (6.0%)	88 (5.4%)
P. malariae	55 (3.1%)	41 (2.5%)
Mixed infection	11 (0.6%)	13 (0.8%)
P. knowlesi	2 (0.1%)	1 (<0.1%)
Unspecified	0 (0.0%)	1 (<0.1%)
Total	**1,792**	**1,618**

Source: Public Health England

Table 2. Cases of malaria in the United Kingdom by geographical distribution: 2017 and 2016

Geographical area (PHE Centre)	2017	2016	% change
London	922	843	9%
West Midlands	161	118	36%
Sout East	155	141	10%
North West	128	107	20%
East of England	114	122	-7%
Yorkshire and Humber	79	68	16%
South West	73	65	12%
East Midlands	50	43	16%
North East	26	22	18%
England total	**1,708**	**1,529**	**12%**
Scotland	50	58	-14%
Wales	24	25	-4%
Northern Ireland	10	6	67%
UK total	**1,792**	**1,618**	

Source: Public Health England

There were six deaths from malaria reported in 2017, the same number as in 2016 and 2015. These were all from *falciparum* malaria acquired in Western Africa (3), Eastern Africa (2) and South-Eastern Asia (1). There is usually a small variation in the number of deaths from malaria in the UK every year but the total for 2017 is in line with the annual average of six over the last ten years. The number of deaths from *vivax* malaria in any year is very low. PHE Malaria Reference Laboratory data over 27 years were combined and demonstrated that older age is a major risk factor for severe *vivax* as well as *falciparum* malaria, with all *vivax* deaths occurring in those aged over 50 years.

During the period 2000–2017, the average age of those who died from *falciparum* malaria was 49 years, reflecting the relatively younger age profile of cases.

Age and sex

Age and sex were known for 1,778/1,792 cases of malaria; of these the majority (67%, 1,188/1,778) were male, consistent with previous years. Males dominated all age groups. The median age was 41 years for males and 40 for females. Children aged less than 18 years accounted for 10% (186) of all cases with known age and sex.

Geographical distribution

London continues to report the largest proportion of cases in England (992/1,708, 58%) with a 9% increase in cases compared to 2016, consistent with the national increase. Of note is the 36% increase in cases reported in the West Midlands compared to 2016 (Table 2).

Travel history and ethnic origin

Of those with information available on travel history, reason for travel and/or country of residence (1,687/1,792, 94%), the majority of malaria cases reported having travelled abroad from the UK (1,221/1,687, 72%). Cases who travelled abroad from the UK include: those where reason for travel was holiday, business/professional, civilian/air crew, armed forces or visiting friends and relatives. The remaining cases were new entrants (also includes UK citizens living abroad and foreign students) accounting for 5% (80/1,687) and foreign visitors to the UK accounting for 5% (79/1,687).

Of the six deaths reported, four were of White British ethnicity, one was of Black African ethnicity and one originated from the Indian subcontinent. Of those with known travel history, three of the cases travelled abroad from the UK, two were new entrants and one was a foreign visitor.

Of the 1,221 cases that travelled abroad from the UK, reason for travel was known for 1,020 (84%). Of these, 814/1,020 (80%) had visited family in their country of origin (also known as visiting friends and relatives, or VFR travellers), 98/1,020 (10%) travelled for business (including armed forces and civilian air crew) and 108/1,020 (11%) travelled for a holiday.

Country/region of birth for cases that travelled abroad from the UK

Country or region of birth information was known for 804 (66%) of 1,221 cases that travelled abroad from the UK, of which almost two-thirds were born in Africa (Figure 1).

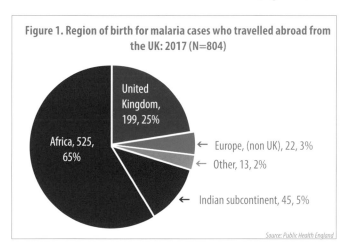

Figure 1. Region of birth for malaria cases who travelled abroad from the UK: 2017 (N=804)

United Kingdom, 199, 25%

Africa, 525, 65%

Europe, (non UK), 22, 3%

Other, 13, 2%

Indian subcontinent, 45, 5%

Source: Public Health England

Table 3: Malaria cases that travelled abroad from the UK by region of birth and proportion of VFR travellers: 2017 (N=740)

Region of birth	N*	VFR*	% VFR
Africa	476	462	97%
Europe – UK	186	75	40%
Indian subcontinent***	44	40	91%
Other****	34	21	62%

*N – cases where region of birth and reason for travel was known

**VFR – cases that have travelled to visit family in country of origin

*** Indian subcontinent here includes: Bangladesh, Bhutan, India, Maldives, Nepal, Pakistan and Sri Lanka

**** includes non UK Europe

Source: Public Health England

Ethnicity for cases that travelled abroad from the UK

Where ethnicity was known, over three-quarters of malaria cases that travelled abroad from the UK were of Black African ethnicity or African descent (76%, 900/1,192) (African descent is determined from country of birth if ethnicity is not given) (Figure 2).

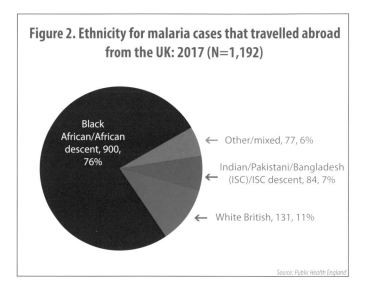

Figure 2. Ethnicity for malaria cases that travelled abroad from the UK: 2017 (N=1,192)

Black African/African descent, 900, 76%

Other/mixed, 77, 6%

Indian/Pakistani/Bangladesh (ISC)/ISC descent, 84, 7%

White British, 131, 11%

Source: Public Health England

Table 4. Cases of malaria that travelled abroad from the UK by species and region of travel: 2017 and 2016

Region of travel	P. falciparum	P. vivax	P. ovale	P. malariae	Mixed	P. knowlesi	2017 total	2016 total
Western Africa	738	–	48	18	6	–	810	638
Eastern Africa	125	4	15	11	–	–	155	147
Middle Africa	84	–	7	3	–	–	94	120
Northern Africa	12	–	–	2	–	–	14	17
Southern Africa	8	–	–	–	–	–	8	3
Africa unspecified	10	1	–	–	–	–	11	6
Southern Asia	2	86	–	1	–	–	89	82
South-Eastern Asia	–	2	–	–	–	2	4	2
Western Asia	–	3	–	–	–	–	3	–
South America	2	4	–	–	–	–	6	3
Caribbean	–	–	–	–	–	–	–	2
Oceania	–	2	–	–	–	–	2	2
Not stated	19	3	2	1	–	–	25	22
Total	**1,000**	**105**	**72**	**36**	**6**	**2**	**1,221**	**1,044**

Source: Public Health England

For non-white British cases, where reason for travel was known, 805/879 (92%) were VFR travellers.

Country/region of travel for cases that travelled from the UK

Table 4 (on the previous page) shows the breakdown of malaria cases reported by region of travel and parasite species. The majority of cases (where travel history was known) continue to be acquired in Africa, with 66% acquired in Western Africa (810/1,221), 13% in Eastern Africa (155/1,221) and 8% in Middle Africa (94/1,221).

While it is important not to over-interpret changes in individual countries because numbers are low, the number of cases acquired in 14 of the top 20 countries increased in 2017 compared to 2016. The largest increases were observed in Nigeria, where there was an increase from 364 cases in 2016 to 470 cases in 2017 (29%), and in Côte d'Ivoire, where the number of cases increased by 75% from 32 in 2016 to 56 in 2017.

There was also a 35% increase in the number of cases in Sierra Leone in 2017 from 91 to 123 cases.

No cryptic cases were reported in 2017.

July 2018

www.publishing.service.gov.uk

Drones vs mosquitoes: fighting malaria in Malawi

Find out how scientists are using drones to help stop the spread of malaria.

By Andrew Brown

KASUNGU, Malawi, 7 September 2018 – In the middle of a muddy field next to a reservoir in north-western Malawi, a team of scientists are hard at work. Boxes of equipment lie scattered around a patch of dry ground, where a scientist programmes an automated drone flight into a laptop perched on a metal box. The craggy peak of Linga Mountain ('watch from afar' in the local language) looms over the lake, casting its reflection in the water.

With a high-pitched whirr of rotor blades, the drone takes off and starts following the shoreline, taking photos as it goes. Once the drone is airborne, the team switch from high-tech to low-tech mode. They collect ladles, rulers and plastic containers and squelch through mud until they reach the water's edge.

The scientists measure the water depth with a ruler and carefully ladle water into the containers. Using a mobile app, they record the GPS location of each sample. Back on dry ground, they count the number of mosquito larvae in each container.

A team from Liverpool School of Tropical Medicine and Lancaster University have been doing the same thing for two weeks at five reservoirs in Kasungu. They are collecting data to identify mosquito breeding sites, so that the larvae can be controlled, reducing the number of adult mosquitoes able to spread malaria.

'Malaria is one of the top three causes of death among children under five years old in Malawi'.

'We stitch together the drone photos to create an aerial map of the reservoir,' says Michelle Stanton, one of the scientists on the team. 'Our water samples tell us where the mosquito breeding sites are, and we can plot these on the map... We can [then] identify the common features of these sites and predict where other breeding sites are.'

Deadly disease

Malaria is a serious issue in Kasungu District and other parts of Malawi. Along with pneumonia and diarrhoea, it is one of the top three causes of death among children under five years old. The disease is preventable and easily treatable if caught early, but if untreated quickly leads to severe complications and death.

Previous efforts to control malaria include distributing bed nets and posting health surveillance assistants in hard to reach areas. These assistants hold regular clinics for children under five and carry rapid diagnostic kits and malaria medication to treat any cases they find. For complicated cases, they provide initial treatment and refer the child to their nearest health facility.

At Kasungu District Hospital, there is a long queue of mothers and children waiting in the morning sunshine outside the Under Five clinic. In a corner of the waiting room, health surveillance assistant Zondiwe Nyirongo sits wearing white plastic gloves and an apron at a desk already littered with used malaria test kits. 'I've done 56 malaria tests so far this morning,' says Zondiwe. 'Of these, 19 were positive. I do up to 300 tests every day, and around half of them are positive.'

One of the children to receive a malaria diagnosis is four-year-old Esther Gama, who arrived with her mother Mary. After the test result, they receive three days' worth of anti-malaria medication. 'Esther is my only child,' she says. 'She's had malaria maybe six or seven times since she turned two years old. I've lost count.'

'Esther got sick three days ago,' Mary says. 'I gave her pain killers but she didn't get better. Then last night she got a fever, so I brought her to the hospital this morning.'

Mary's calm exterior is somewhat deceptive. 'I do worry about malaria a lot,' she admits. 'Several children in our village have been admitted to hospital with serious cases. Some of them died.'

'I do up to 300 tests every day, and around half of them are positive.'

Malaria is the number one cause of hospital admissions and deaths among children under five in the district. The fatalities are usually caused by people bringing their children to hospital too late.

'We lack resources such as blood supplies for transfusions,' says Liz Msowoya, the Kasunga District Medical Officer. 'There is also a high HIV rate in this area so relatives cannot always donate blood. Sometimes the health workers donate their own blood because they don't want the child to die. But other times there is nothing we can do.'

Innovative approach

Chris Jones from the Malawi Liverpool Wellcome Trust Centre, who is co-leading the drone project with Michelle, says that existing anti-malaria measures like health surveillance assistants and mosquito nets have led to a dramatic decrease in deaths over the last two decades, but that to reduce this further, new tactics are needed.

'This is the first time the drones approach has been tried,' he says. 'If we can prove the concept, this could become another malaria prevention measure to be used alongside bed nets and village health workers.'

The project made use of Unicef Malawi's Humanitarian Drone Testing Corridor. Launched in 2017 with the Government of Malawi, this allows universities, companies and individuals to conduct test flights within an 80-km diameter area centred on Kasungu airfield. Tests must have a humanitarian or development application in the areas of transport, imagery or connectivity, and provide training opportunities for local Malawians.

As well as securing permission to fly, Unicef has conducted community sensitisation activities in the corridor, so that local people know what drones are, and what they are doing.

Michelle says that her mosquito project would not have been possible without Unicef's drone corridor. 'Our contacts are in the health sector, not civil aviation,' she explains. 'It would have been very difficult for us to get permission to fly and conduct the community sensitisation ourselves. With the drone corridor, however, we could just come in and fly straight away.'

6 September 2018

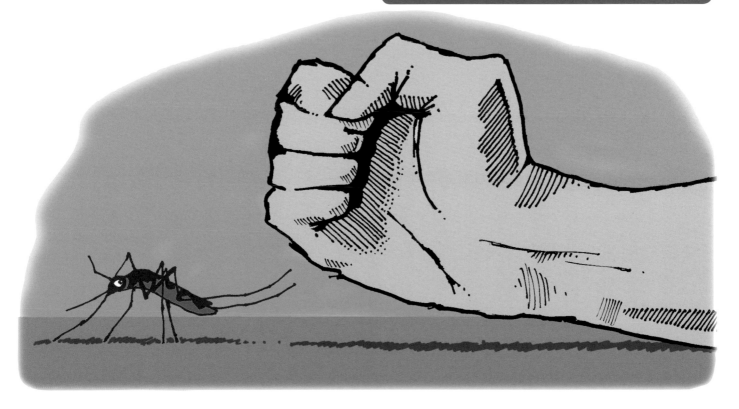

Immunisation

A record 123 million children were immunized globally in 2017 but millions of children are still not reached by potentially life-saving vaccines.

Immunisation is one of the most cost-effective public health interventions to date, averting an estimated two to three million deaths every year. As a direct result of immunisation, the world is closer than ever to eradicating polio, with only three remaining polio endemic countries – Afghanistan, Nigeria and Pakistan. Children under five deaths from measles, a major child killer, declined by 85 per cent worldwide and by 89 per cent in sub-Saharan Africa between 2000 and 2016. And as of March 2018, all but 14 countries have eliminated maternal and neonatal tetanus, a disease with a fatality rate of 70 to 100 per cent among newborns. The percentage of children receiving the diphtheria, tetanus and pertussis vaccine (DTP) is often used as an indicator of how well countries are providing routine immunisation services. In 2017, global coverage rates for the third dose of the diphtheria, tetanus and pertussis vaccine (DTP3) reached 85 per cent, up from 72 per cent in 2000 and 21 per cent in 1980. Still, progress has stalled over the current decade, and 71 countries have yet to achieve the Global Vaccine Action Plan (GVAP) target of 90 per cent or greater coverage of DTP3. 19.9 million children under one year of age worldwide did not receive the three recommended doses of DTP in 2017, and 20.8 million children in the same age group had failed to receive a single dose of measles-containing vaccine.

Conflict is one of the main factors – along with under-investments in national immunisation programmes, vaccine stock-outs and disease outbreaks – disrupting health systems and preventing sustainable delivery of vaccination services. About 40 per cent (almost eight million) of the of the under-immunised infants live in fragile or humanitarian settings, including countries affected by conflicts. These children are the most vulnerable to disease outbreaks. In Yemen, for example, children accounted for over 58 per cent of the more than one million people affected by a cholera outbreak or watery diarrhoea in 2017 alone.

To achieve 90% DTP3 coverage, vaccinations in 71 countries must be accelerated

In 2017, ten countries had less than 50 per cent coverage for DTP3 or the first dose of measles containing vaccine (MCV1), many of which are fragile states and affected by emergencies: Angola, Central African Republic, Chad, Equatorial Guinea, Guinea, Nigeria, Somalia, South Sudan, Syrian Arab Republic and Ukraine. But more than half of all children unvaccinated for DTP3 lived in just five countries: Nigeria, India, Pakistan, Indonesia and Ethiopia. Note that populous developing countries may contribute significantly to the number of unvaccinated children despite achieving relatively high rates of immunisation coverage. Efforts to raise global immunisation levels will require a strong focus on the countries where the highest numbers of unvaccinated children live – while also ensuring that countries where children are most likely to miss out on immunisation are not neglected.

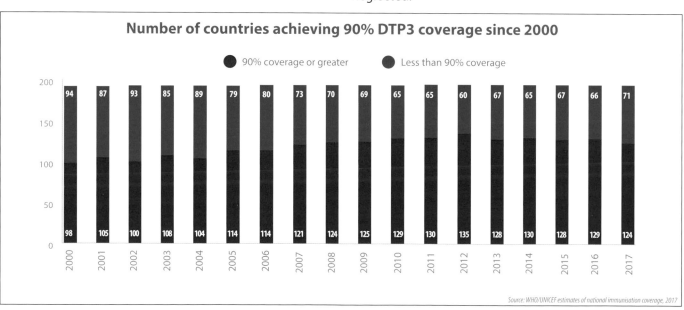

Number of countries achieving 90% DTP3 coverage since 2000

● 90% coverage or greater   ● Less than 90% coverage

Year	90% coverage or greater	Less than 90% coverage
2000	94	98
2001	87	105
2002	93	100
2003	85	108
2004	89	104
2005	79	114
2006	80	114
2007	73	121
2008	70	124
2009	69	125
2010	65	129
2011	65	130
2012	60	135
2013	67	128
2014	65	130
2015	67	128
2016	66	129
2017	71	124

Source: WHO/UNICEF estimates of national immunisation coverage, 2017

Coverage challenges persist in fragile states and those affected by conflict

Through Unicef's joint efforts with partners and countries, vaccines have become safer and more accessible than ever before. The cost of fully immunising children in low-income countries is just US$18 per child, down from US$24.5 in 2013. An increasing number of countries are now offering pneumococcal conjugate vaccine (134 countries as of end of 2017) and rotavirus vaccine (90 countries as of end of 2017) in their immunisation programmes, thus offering protection against pneumonia and diarrhoea. Human papillomavirus (HPV) is the most common viral infection of the reproductive tract, and can cause cervical cancer in women. In 2017, the HPV vaccine was introduced in 79 countries. Use of underutilised vaccines, such as those against yellow fever and Japanese encephalitis, has also been expanded. However, while low-income countries have largely been able to close coverage gaps with assistance from Gavi, the Vaccine Alliance, vaccine introduction is lagging in middle-income countries who struggle to find both national resources and external funding sources.

No child should die from a preventable cause, and all children should be able to reach their full potential in health and well-being. The cost of a vaccine, often less than US$1, is much lower than the cost of treating a sick child or fighting a disease outbreak. Each US$1 invested in childhood vaccination produces a return on investment of US$44 in low- and middle-income countries.

July 2018

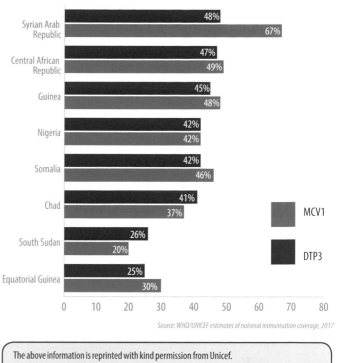

Coverage challenges persist in fragile states and those affected by conflict

DTP3 and MCV1 coverage in countries with less than 50 per cent coverage of DTP3, 2017

Country	MCV1	DTP3
Syrian Arab Republic	48%	67%
Central African Republic	47%	49%
Guinea	45%	48%
Nigeria	42%	42%
Somalia	42%	46%
Chad	41%	37%
South Sudan	26%	20%
Equatorial Guinea	25%	30%

Source: WHO/UNICEF estimates of national immunisation coverage, 2017

www.unicef.org

Onions could hold key to fighting antibiotic resistance

A type of onion could help the fight against antibiotic resistance in cases of tuberculosis, a UCL and Birkbeck-led study suggests.

Researchers believe the antibacterial properties extracted from the Persian shallot could increase the effects of existing antibiotic treatment.

The study, published in *Scientific Reports*, was led by Dr Sanjib Bhakta of Birkbeck, University of London and UCL's Professor Simon Gibbons, who worked with a team of scientists from Birkbeck, UCL, the University of Greenwich, the University of East London and Royal Free Hospital.

When a patient has a bacterial infection, they may be prescribed an antibiotic. In the case of TB, they will likely be prescribed a cocktail of four antibiotics including Isoniazid and Rifampicin – but increasingly, the pathogens in bacterial infections are developing resistance to antibiotic drugs.

This means the drug loses its ability to effectively control or kill harmful bacteria and is free to grow and cause further damage to the patient, which can be passed along to the population at large. Therefore, there is a pressing need to develop new classes of antibacterials to combat antibiotic resistance, which this research may help progress.

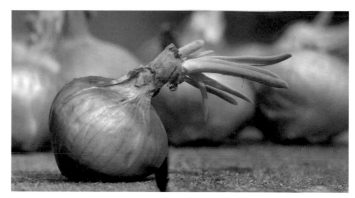

The team investigated extracts of bulbs from *Allium Stipitatum* – also known as the Persian shallot and used as a staple part of Iranian cooking – and its antibacterial effects. They synthesised the chemical compounds present in these plants in order to better understand and optimise their antibacterial potential.

They tested four different synthesised compounds, all of which showed a significant reduction in the presence of the bacteria in the multidrug-resistant tuberculosis – the most promising candidate of which, with highest therapeutic index, inhibited growth of the isolated TB cells by more than 99.9%.

The team concluded that the chemical compounds may work as templates for the discovery of new drug treatment to combat strains of tuberculosis, which have previously developed resistance to anti-bacterial drugs.

Dr Bhakta, of Birkbeck's Department of Biological Sciences, said: 'Despite a concerted global effort to prevent the spread of tuberculosis, approximately ten million new cases and two million deaths were reported in 2016. As many as 50 million people worldwide are currently infected with multi-drug resistant TB, which means it's vital to develop new antibacterials.

'In searching for new antibacterials, we tend to focus on molecules that are potent enough to be developed commercially as new drug entities by themselves. However, in this study we show that by inhibiting the key intrinsic resistance properties of the TB, one could increase the effects of existing antibiotic treatment and reverse the tide of already existing drug resistance.'

Professor Gibbons, Head of UCL Pharmaceutical and Biological Chemistry, said: 'Natural products from plants and microbes have enormous potential as a source of new antibiotics. Nature is an amazingly creative chemist and it is likely that plants such as the Persian shallot produce these chemicals as a defence against microbes in their environment. Dr Bhakta and I will be dedicating our research to discovering new antibiotics and understanding how they function. We believe that nature holds the key for new antibiotic chemotypes.'

22 January 2018

Antibiotic-resistant superbugs 'will kill 90,000 Britons by 2050'

OECD says superbugs could kill 1.3 million people in Europe unless more is done to tackle issue.

More than 90,000 people in Britain will die over the next three decades unless action is taken to halt the rise in antibiotic-resistant superbug infections, a report has warned.

The Organisation for Economic Co-operation and Development (OECD) estimates resistant infections could kill about 2.4 million people in Europe, North America and Australia by 2050 unless more is done to tackle the problem, which it describes as 'one of the biggest threats to modern medicine'.

This includes about 1.3 million deaths in Europe and 90,000 in Britain.

Simple hygiene measures such as hand washing and more conservative prescribing of antibiotics could prevent some of the deaths, the authors said. The report said enhanced rapid testing to ensure patients are given appropriate drugs could also help overcome the looming crisis.

There are growing concerns about the increasing number of infections that have evolved resistance to first-line drugs, leaving a dwindling number of treatment options available. The problem of resistance is growing even more rapidly in low- and middle-income countries.

The report warns that southern Europe risks being particularly affected, with Italy, Greece and Portugal forecast to top the list of OECD countries with the highest mortality rates from antimicrobial resistance.

Resistance to second- and third-line antibiotics – used as backup to treat infections when common antibiotics do not work – is expected to increase over the coming decades it says.

The report comes after health officials in England launched a campaign to try to prevent people from asking for the drugs when they do not need them.

Public Health England said antibiotics were essential for treating serious bacterial infections but the drugs were frequently being prescribed for coughs, sore throats and earache, which usually improve without the medication.

Tim Jinks, head of the Wellcome Trust's drug-resistant infections priority programme, said: 'This new OECD report offers important insight into how simple, cost-effective surveillance, prevention and control methods could save lives globally.

'Drug-resistant superbugs are on the rise worldwide and represent a fundamental threat to global health and development. This report provides yet further evidence that investing to tackle the problem now will save lives and deliver big payoffs in the future.'

A short-term investment to tackle superbugs would save lives and money, the OECD said, estimating that halting the rise of resistant infections would cost just $2 (£1.50) per person a year. The health body's latest campaign reminds people that if they are feeling unwell 'antibiotics aren't always needed'.

7 November 2018

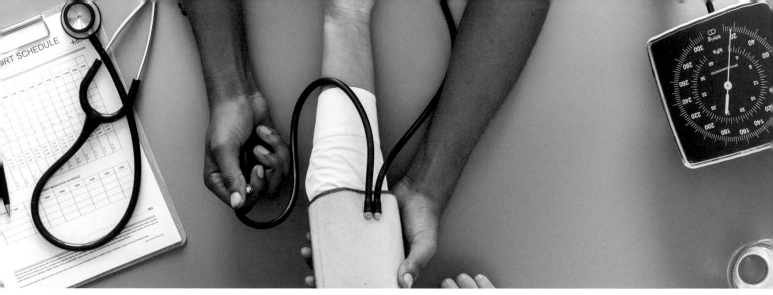

The flat-pack clinic that could revolutionise healthcare in isolated communities

By Sarah Newey, global health security correspondent

Doctors working in remote parts of the world are often forced to operate out of flimsy tents or repurposed buildings which can be cramped, unhygienic and not fit for purpose.

But now an innovative temporary clinic, which could 'revolutionise' healthcare outreach programmes around the world, has been unveiled.

The Global Clinic, designed for the charity Doctors of the World, is a portable plywood structure which offers doctors a clean, safe, soundproof environment to treat patients.

The structures – whose components are slotted together in a similar way to a piece of flat-pack furniture – are easy to transport and can be adapted to suit conditions on the ground.

'Often we're working with tents in emergency situations, for instance with the refugee crisis which exploded in 2015,' Ellen Waters, director of development at Doctors of the World, told *The Telegraph*.

'But the type of work we do needs something more private, more secure, more clinical - and of course tents are unhygienic. They can get very muddy and are not a nice environment to be in,' she said.

The innovative design was created by architects Rogers Stirk Harbour + Partners and engineers BuroHappold Engineering and ChapmanBDSP. It will be on display at the Wellcome Collection until April, as part of an exhibition exploring the relationship between architecture and health.

The lightweight structure, which takes about a day to erect, weighs just 400kg making it easily transportable. The plans can be emailed to a computer anywhere in the world, with the components being manufactured locally.

'We wanted to rethink temporary clinics, to give doctors a clean environment to work in,' said Ivan Harbour, architect and senior partner at Rogers Stirk Harbour.

'Rather than fabricating and exporting a finished product, the design data [plans] can be sent around the world and the cutting can happen in the nearest available place. Communities can then be involved in the assembly and given ownership of the space,' he said.

The prototype on show in London cost £4,000 to manufacture and construct. But Mr Harbour told *The Telegraph* that the price would be 'considerably lower' in other regions, where labour and materials are cheaper.

'These structures would absolutely revolutionise our work,' said Ms Waters. 'They would be quick to deploy, and would allow us to provide doctors and patients with a comfortable environment to be in, despite the climate.'

The plywood structure's outer skin could be adapted according to climate – from a waterproof tarpaulin in cold, damp regions like Eastern Europe, to a breathable mesh in Africa.

Another key element of the design is its soundproofing, enabling doctors to conduct consultations privately.

The clinic on display is the result of two years' planning and development, and Doctors of the World hope that the design could be rolled out within the next 18 months, following trials in the field and fundraising.

'Now that it's got to this point and it's on show, there's a buzz and excitement around our community,' Pete Aldridge, fundraising manager at Doctors of the World, told *The Telegraph*.

'There has been a lot of interest in being the first to have one.'

3 October 2018

Keep Antibiotics Working campaign returns

New data shows that over three million surgeries and cancer treatments may become life threatening without antibiotics.

The 'Keep Antibiotics Working' campaign returns to alert the public to the risks of antibiotic resistance, urging them to always take their doctor, nurse or healthcare professional's advice on antibiotics.

Antibiotics are a vital tool used to manage infections. Public Health England's (PHE's) *English Surveillance Programme for Antimicrobial Utilisation and Resistance (ESPAUR)* report published Tuesday, 23 October 2018, highlights how more than three million common procedures such as cesarean sections and hip replacements could become life-threatening without them.

Without antibiotics, infections related to surgery could double, putting people at risk of dangerous complications. Cancer patients are also much more vulnerable if antibiotics don't work; both cancer and the treatment (chemotherapy) reduce the ability of the immune system to fight infections. Antibiotics are critical to both prevent and treat infections in these patients.

Antibiotics are essential to treat serious bacterial infections, but they are frequently being used to treat illnesses such as coughs, earache and sore throats that can get better by themselves. Taking antibiotics encourages harmful bacteria that live inside you to become resistant. That means that antibiotics may not work when you really need them.

The threat of antibiotic resistance continues to grow. Bloodstream infections have increased and the report shows that antibiotic-resistant bloodstream infections rose by an estimated 35% between 2013 and 2017.

Despite the risks of antibiotic resistance, research shows that 38% of people still expect an antibiotic from a doctor's surgery, NHS walk-in centre or 'GP out-of-hours' service when they visited with a cough, flu or a throat, ear, sinus or chest infection in 2017.

The 'Keep Antibiotics Working' campaign educates the public about the risks of antibiotic resistance, urging people to always take healthcare professionals' advice as to when they need antibiotics. The campaign also provides effective self-care advice to help individuals and their families feel better if they are not prescribed antibiotics.

Professor Paul Cosford, Medical Director, Public Health England said:

'Antibiotics are an essential part of modern medicine, keeping people safe from infection when they are at their most vulnerable. It's concerning that, in the not too distant future, we may see more cancer patients, mothers who've had caesareans and patients who've had other surgery facing life-threatening situations if antibiotics fail to ward off infections.

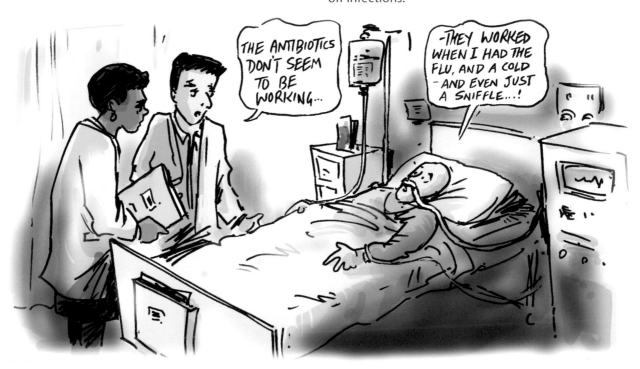

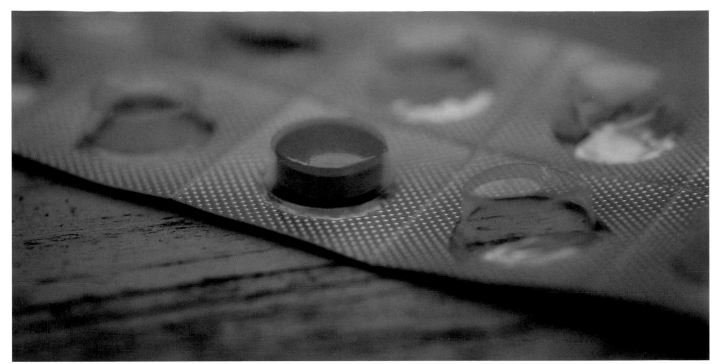

'We need to preserve antibiotics for when we really need them and we are calling on the public to join us in tackling antibiotic resistance by listening to your GP, pharmacist or nurse's advice and only taking antibiotics when necessary. Taking antibiotics just in case may seem like a harmless act, but it can have grave consequences for you and your family's health in future.'

Professor Dame Sally Davies, Chief Medical Officer for England said:

'The evidence is clear that without swift action to reduce infections, we are at risk of putting medicine back in the dark ages – to an age where common procedures we take for granted could become too dangerous to perform, and treatable conditions become life-threatening.

'The UK has made great efforts in recent years to reduce prescribing rates of antibiotics; however, there continues to be a real need to preserve the drugs we have so that they remain effective for those who really need them and prevent infections emerging in the first place. This is not just an issue for doctors and nurses, the public have a huge role to play – today's data and the launch of the national 'Keep Antibiotics Working' campaign must be a further wake-up call to us all.'

Professor Helen Stokes-Lampard, Chair of the Royal College of GPs, said:

'GPs are already doing an excellent job at reducing antibiotics prescriptions, but we often come under considerable pressure from patients to prescribe them.

'We need to get to a stage where antibiotics are not seen as a "catch all" for every illness or a "just in case" backup option – and patients need to understand that if their doctor doesn't prescribe antibiotics it's because they genuinely believe they are not the most appropriate course of treatment.

'It's crucial that we continue to get this message out, which is why we're pleased to support Public Health England's "Keep Antibiotics Working" campaign to make sure we can carry on delivering safe, effective care to our patients both now and in the future.'

Background

1. The Ipsos MORI Capibus Survey, 'Attitudes towards antibiotics, 2017' was conducted between 24 January to 5 February 2017 with a representative sample size of 1,691 adults (aged 15+) in England only. 269 contacted a health professional with a respiratory tract infection in the last year – these participants were asked: 'What did you expect from the doctor's surgery, walk-in centre, urgent or out of hours with your cough, throat, ear, sinus, chest infection or flu?'

2. The campaign will run from Tuesday 23 October 2018 across England for eight weeks and will be supported with advertising, partnerships with local pharmacies and GP surgeries, and social media activity.

3. The campaign is part of a wider cross-government strategy to help preserve antibiotics. The Government's *UK Five Year Antimicrobial Resistance Strategy 2013 to 2018* set out aims to improve the knowledge and understanding of AMR, conserve and steward the effectiveness of existing treatments, and stimulate the development of new antibiotics, diagnostics and novel therapies.

23 October 2018

www.gov.uk

Monitor lizard venom could be used to treat human blood clots

An article from The Conversation.

THE CONVERSATION

By Kevin Arbuckle, Lecturer in Biosciences, Swansea University

To be venomous, an animal – or plant, or even bacterium – must have a toxic secretion and a mechanism for delivering it into another animal, in order to feed or defend itself. Venoms tend to be highly complex mixtures of molecules containing both toxins and non-toxic components, and much research has gone into understanding the composition of venoms from many different species.

Because venoms are essentially pools of molecules that have evolved to alter the physiology of other animals – whether they be predators or prey – they are excellent candidates for the development of new medicinal drugs. This follows from the fact that most physiological systems are carefully balanced at some optimal point. For instance, if blood pressure is too high, a person will suffer hypertension, but if it is too low they will suffer from hypotension.

Some animal venoms have evolved to quickly decrease blood pressure, which can cause shock in a prey animal and immobilise it so it can be eaten. However, if we can identify the toxins which lead to the drop in blood pressure, we can perhaps use them to lower blood pressure in people with hypertension. The highly variable nature of venom between, and even within, species means that there are a great many potential drugs out there.

Kill or cure

The development of drugs from venoms has already proven successful in the past. At least six venom-derived drugs are currently on the market in the US. Perhaps the best known example is the drug Capoten, which is derived from a South American species of pit viper, *Bothrops jararaca*. Capoten is an ACE inhibitor medication (which block the body from producing a chemical called angiotensin II, which in turn narrows the blood vessels) that is used to treat conditions such as hypertension.

Similarly, the drug Byetta is derived from the venom of the Gila monster (*Heloderma suspectum*), a venomous lizard. Byetta is used to treat type 2 diabetes: it increases insulin secretion by the pancreas, and slows glucose absorption in the gut. Together, this lowers blood sugar levels and reduces appetite.

Monitor lizards – a group which includes the famous Komodo dragon – have traditionally not been considered to have venom. However, recent work has suggested that they are indeed venomous, based on the presence of sophisticated glands in the lower jaw, which produce similar toxins to those found in other lizards and snakes known to be venomous.

Nevertheless, some biologists have disagreed with these findings, in part arguing that the 'venom' is not important to these lizards for their predation or defence. But our new paper has contributed more data that suggests that not only are these lizards venomous, but that they may have toxins which have potential to treat blood disorders in humans.

Toxins and drug development

For our research, we examined 16 species of monitor lizard species and found that all had venoms which contained toxins similar to some of those found in venomous snakes and Gila monsters.

In addition, each species had a different subset of toxins. This suggests that natural selection is actively favouring diversification of the toxins, and that these molecules are doing something important to the lizard's evolutionary fitness.

We also demonstrated that – in addition to effects previously documented from monitor lizard venom – at least some venoms can cause muscle spasms, and all the venoms destroyed the blood's clotting ability.

The effects that lizard venom has on the blood is due to toxins which cleave – damage by 'cutting' – fibrinogen, which is necessary for clot formation. We found that how quickly fibrinogen was cleaved, and which parts of fibrinogen were affected, varied between monitor lizard species. This means that there are several different varieties of toxins which contribute to stopping blood from clotting. In prey, this would quickly cause loss of blood, resulting in weakness and shock.

As many human medical conditions are caused by blood clots occurring where it shouldn't, such as many heart attacks, strokes and thromboses, lizard venom could potentially be a treasure trove of previously unexplored toxins that stop blood clots from happening. As the idea of venom in monitor lizards has been previously disregarded, we now have the opportunity to develop new drugs from the toxins in monitor lizard venom to treat blood clotting disorders.

The existence of any drugs that may arise from these venoms is still many years off, but it just goes to show that medicines can come from the unlikeliest of sources – and that future studies on monitor lizard venom may bring large benefits for us all.

21 August 2017

www.theconversation.com

UK response to Ebola cases in the DRC

The UK Government is working with the government of DRC and World Health Organization (WHO) following the confirmation of two cases of the disease in May.

The UK Government is working with the government of the Democratic Republic of the Congo (DRC) and World Health Organization (WHO) to monitor the situation and be ready to act quickly to tackle the spread of the disease.

International Development Secretary Penny Mordaunt said:

'The Ebola epidemic in 2014 highlighted that to save lives we need to act quickly to stop the spread of this disease.

'We're well-practised in responding to disease outbreaks, and are coordinating across government to support the WHO in their leadership of the response. Vaccines have been stockpiled, we have built research and monitoring capacity, and the Rapid Support Team of health experts stand ready to be deployed if needed.

'I've spoken to the UK team in the DRC and heard how we are working with the country's government, the WHO and other partners to monitor the situation closely and to take fast and appropriate action to tackle the spread of Ebola, to keep us all safe from this disease.

'I'd also like to thank the brave healthcare experts already working on this response, and on broader work to tackle disease outbreaks across the globe to stop these threats reaching our shores.'

It is vital we are ready to respond rapidly when outbreaks are detected, which is why the UK is the second largest contributor to the WHO's Contingency Fund for Emergencies, from which $1 million has already been mobilised to respond to this outbreak. We also work to strengthen health systems in high-risk countries such as DRC, so that they can better detect and tackle disease outbreaks when they arise.

DFID and Wellcome jointly fund a research initiative on epidemic preparedness. Today, DFID is making available £1 million from this programme to support the rapid response, in addition to a further £2 million being made available by Wellcome.

DFID has worked with Wellcome to develop a safe vaccine for Ebola which is currently stockpiled, ready for use, by the Global Vaccines Alliance, GAVI – to which we are a major contributor.

The UK Public Health Rapid Support Team is also on standby ready to be deployed to support the response, if required.

DRC has experienced several Ebola outbreaks since 1976, and the country is familiar with managing the disease.

The FCO have also updated travel advice for DFID DRC.

10 May 2018

www.gov.uk

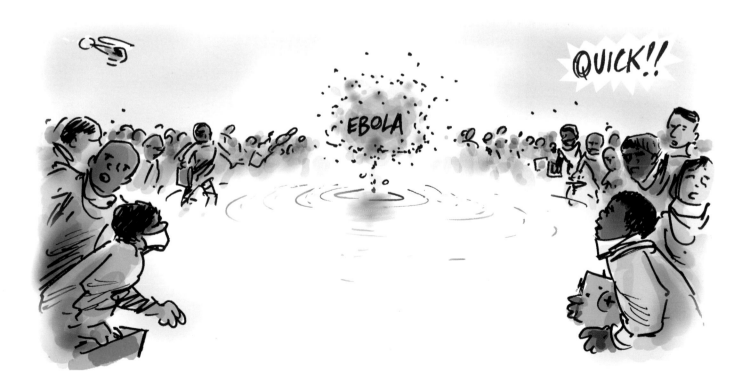

How will new technologies change what you do?

By Samir Prakash and Liz Talbot

Novel technology is bringing many opportunities and disruptions. These offer possibilities that could change our lives, from what public services are offered to how we move around the world.

The Government Office for Science's Emerging Technology Programme helps government think about how potential new technologies may affect policy choices. The Programme scans for and assesses novel technologies emerging from all areas of science and engineering. Medicine is one area in which many important new technologies have been identified. This is the first in a series of blog posts that covers some of the innovative and exciting technologies the scan has brought to our attention.

Medicine's new frontier in technology

The UK is a global leader in medical technologies and has recently made some significant commitments to technological advances that will help reshape healthcare and offer us all a healthier future. The UK has signalled its commitment to remaining a world leader with ventures such as the 100,000 Genomes Project, the Organ-on-a-Chip Technologies Network and a Life Sciences Sector Deal. Below are three emerging technologies identified by GOS' Emerging Technology Scan that could change how we practise medicine in the UK.

Organs-on-a-chip

From beating hearts to breathing lungs, organs-on-a-chip may become some of the hottest new tools for biomedical research. Scientists have created working models for a range of organs, including the liver, the kidneys and even an eye – complete with blinking eyelid. Researchers intend to use these devices to model disease and facilitate drug development, replacing animal testing and carrying out personalised medicine in a more effective way. For example, rather than use generic cell lines to study the effects of drugs, doctors in the future could use cells from the patient to test how they would react to different treatment options. This would allow more targeted and effective therapies. The technology is still in its infancy, but what was once inconceivable – risk-free biomedical testing on living human organs – has moved a step closer.

Genomic vaccines

Vaccines teach the immune system to recognise antigens – proteins on the surface of a pathogen – and develop an immune response to them. They do this by either delivering a dead or weakened form of the pathogen, or just its associated antigens, into the body. A new kind of vaccine may fundamentally change that. Genomic vaccines comprise DNA or RNA that encode the target antigens directly. Once injected, the genetic material enters cells and causes the production of the antigens, triggering the desired immune

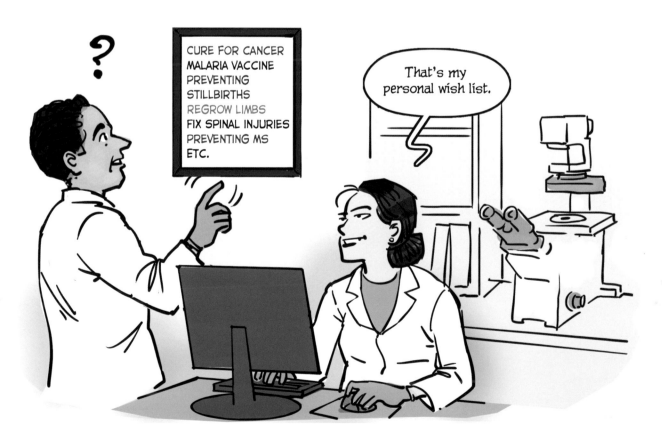

response. Genomic vaccines offer many advantages: they are quicker to manufacture than traditional vaccines and can be produced rapidly when a more virulent strain of a virus like Zika or Ebola suddenly emerges. A single such vaccine can include code for multiple antigens, protecting a person from several diseases, and they can be readily changed if a pathogen mutates. Worldwide, clinical trials are underway for avian flu, Zika, Ebola, hepatitis C, HIV and some cancers. These vaccines may change the way we tackle infectious diseases.

Liquid biopsies

A major goal of cancer research is to detect cancers at an early stage – before symptoms are apparent – when treating them is likely to be easier and more successful. Liquid biopsies promise to do just that. Liquid biopsies use advanced gene sequencing technologies to detect cancer DNA in blood samples. They are currently used to aid in treatment decisions for those already diagnosed with certain types of cancer, but they have potential far beyond that. Traditional tissue biopsies do not examine the whole tumour, and so may miss cells with more dangerous mutations. In principle, liquid biopsy can detect the full spectrum of mutations and so indicate if more aggressive treatment is necessary. In future, they may provide a simple screening test for early diagnosis of cancer in people who seem perfectly healthy. While it is still early days for liquid biopsies, researchers are hopeful that they will fulfil their potential – and usher in an era of personalised cancer treatment

6 September 2018

There's a test that shows doctors if antibiotics will work or not – so why isn't it being used?

THE CONVERSATION

An article from The Conversation.

By Peter Lambert, Professor of Microbial Chemistry, Aston University

It is estimated that antibiotics add an average of 20 years to all of our lives. However, their overuse, misuse and inappropriate use has encouraged microbes to evolve resistance, resulting in the emergence of untreatable 'superbugs' that threaten the basis of modern medicine.

Drug-resistant infections are already responsible for more than half a million deaths worldwide each year, estimated to rise to over 10 million by 2050. Antimicrobial resistance must be managed with the utmost urgency and careful stewardship of antibiotics can help conserve antibiotics for future generations.

One of the big problems is that antibiotics are routinely prescribed for infections where they simply won't work. If you have a virus such as cold or flu, you feel bad and would like the doctor to give you antibiotics because many of us believe they can fix everything. Your doctor wants to help

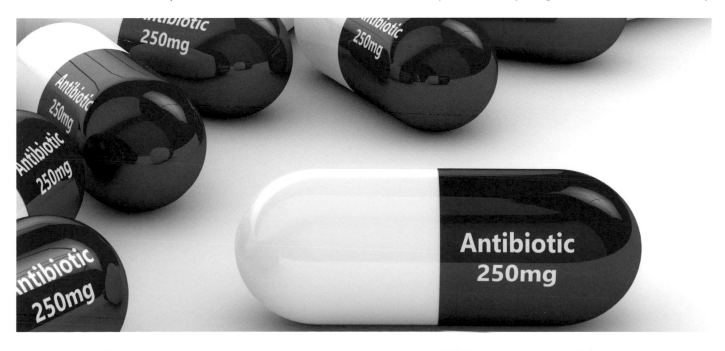

too and has a busy workload so they prescribe them. But this exacerbates the problem because it builds resistance in a population. It has been suggested that 10% of the 34 million antibiotics prescribed in the UK every year are given to people who don't need them. In the US, this may be as high as 30%.

Respiratory tract infections (RTIs), such as cold and flu and pneumonia, affect the throat, chest (airways and lungs) and sinuses. While they are most often caused by viruses (where antibiotics do not help), they can also be caused by bacteria (where antibiotics help). Given that RTIs are one of the main reasons why people visit their GP or pharmacist, developing a good way of telling between the two is crucial to cutting inappropriate prescriptions.

The £10 million Longitude Prize, introduced in 2014, aims to reward the development of new diagnostic tests that can help to guide the effective use of antibiotics and avoid their inappropriate use. Rapid, affordable, easy-to-use tests that indicate the presence of a bacterial infection used at a GP clinic, for example, would allow more targeted use of antibiotics, and an overall reduction in misdiagnosis and

prescription. But there is some reason to think that not enough is being done to make use of these tests.

Take the diagnosis of pneumonia. There is convincing evidence that measurement of a C-reactive protein (CRP) in the blood, which increases in the body when there is inflammation caused by infection, can help GPs determine whether or not a person with symptoms of a chest infection has pneumonia and should be treated with antibiotics.

In 2014, NICE, the UK health watchdog, recommended that GPs should consider carrying out a CRP blood test on patients with symptoms of lower respiratory tract infection. It said that if, after a clinical assessment, a diagnosis of pneumonia cannot be made and it's unclear whether antibiotics should be prescribed, the test should be carried out.

17 February 2017

Brexit risk: more than a quarter of midwives at some London hospitals are EU nationals

By Andy Jones

More than a quarter of midwives in some London maternity units are from the European Union, new analysis reveals, while recruitment from the continent has plummeted since the Brexit vote.

Sixteen hospital trusts in the capital currently rely on the EU for more than 10% of their midwives, shows the most recent data from NHS Digital (see table opposite. And at two trusts – University College Hospitals (UCL) and North Middlesex University Hospital – more than a quarter of midwives are EU nationals.

Meanwhile just 33 midwives arrived from the European Economic Area (EEA) in the last year up to March 2018, which was a fall of nearly 90% from the year before the referendum, according to data from the Nursing and Midwifery Council. Over the same period, 234 EEA midwives left their posts. This drastic decline is sharpening an existing staffing crisis, with 3,500 midwife posts currently empty.

The referendum result has a major impact on recruitment, according to Danny Mortimer, chief executive of NHS Employers. 'We have absolutely seen applications from within the EU drop,' he said. 'Just plummet. Graphs show EU nurses arriving up until the referendum and within six months, it just drops like a stone.'

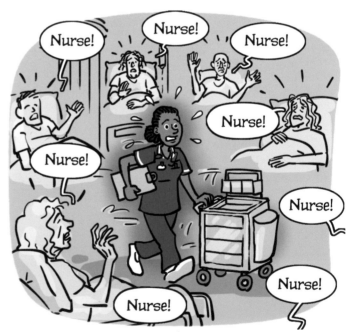

Brexit has put hospital recruiters in a difficult position, he added. 'NHS employers haven't known what to say when going out to recruit as they don't know the implications in terms of EU staff's migration status.'

UCL has stopped attempting to recruit from Europe despite having a vacancy rate of 9% across all clinical staff, it told

Trust	Proportion of midwives who are EU nationals
University College London Hospitals NHS Foundation Trust	26%
North Middlesex Universtiy Hospital NHS Trust	26%
Guy's and St Thomas' NHS Foundation Trust	19%
Whittington Health NHS Trust	18%
Homerton University Hospital NHS Foundation Trust	18
Imperial College Healthcare NHS Trust	18%
Hillingdon Hospitals NHS Foundation Trust	17%
Chelsea and Westminster Hospital NHS Foundation Trust	16%
Barts Health NHS Trust	16%
St George's University Hospitals NHS Foundation Trust	15%
Barking, Havering and Redbridge University Hospitals NHS Trust	14%
Kingston Hospital NHS Foundation Trust	12
Ashford and St. Peter's Hospitals NHS Foundation Trust	12%
Royal Free London NHS Foundation Trust	12%
Croydon Health Services NHS Trust	12%
Epsom and St Helier University Hospitals NHS Trust	11%
Lewisham and Greenwich NHS Trust	10%

Source: The Bureau of Investigative Journalism

the Bureau, because 'interest in coming to the UK appears to have declined.'

'A campaign to a mainland EU nation would only prove cost-effective for us if we recruited an intake of at least 15–20 candidates,' the spokesperson said.

Brexit is not the only factor driving the EU recruitment crisis, said Mortimer. A weak pound, London's high cost of living and new language testing brought in by the Government in 2016 have all put people off.

'We have seen a definite drop in the number of staff applying for jobs from European countries.'

The overall picture of EU staff recruitment and retention is complex. Some London units highlighted that the number of EU midwives included a high percentage of Irish staff, who it is thought are more likely to remain in posts after Brexit than their counterparts from mainland Europe, because of Ireland and the UK's shared values and lifestyle.

The strategic director of one London trust told us that his team had consciously stopped recruiting in the EU as European nurses and midwives only tended to stay around two years. Many arrived so they could gain experience in high-quality hospitals or for the life experience, but then – when faced with raising a family or setting down roots – returned home because of UK living costs or personal choice. The trust had particular success hiring nurses from the Philippines and India as they typically stayed longer.

Retaining midwives is a particular problem. Despite more than 2,000 people graduating in midwifery per year, the total number of midwives in England rose by just 67 in the last 12-month period, because of the amount of people leaving the profession. 'We seem to need 30 graduates just to add the equivalent of one full-time NHS midwife,' said the latest *State of Maternity Services* report by the Royal College of Midwives.

The Government has previously said it is 'publicly committed to the EU Settlement Scheme which will allow any EU citizen currently residing in the UK to register to remain here indefinitely, with broadly the same rights as now.'

Such a promise does not appear to have reassured EU midwives and nurses that are already in England, or those considering joining the NHS. The Nursing and Midwifery Council (NMC) register shows new arrivals from the EEA fell by 88% between 2015/16 (the year before the Brexit referendum) and 2017/18, while the number leaving the register increased by a nearly a third.

Half of the EEA nationals leaving the register said that 'Brexit has encouraged me to consider working outside the UK,' according to the NMC.

It's less than ten months since the NHS emerged from the worst winter crisis on record. To take just one marker as an example, from December 2017 to March 2018 there were more trolley waits of more than four hours than the total amount in the same months from 2010 to 2014 combined.

On Monday, trade association NHS Providers said this winter would be even tougher. It highlighted the major role staff shortages have in driving this crisis, with a 'double negative effect' – services cannot be expanded to the extent needed and existing staff are put under much greater pressure.

'Historically the UK has always relied on international recruitment to address domestic supply problems,' the report pointed out, warning that the decision to leave the EU combined with new language tests introduced in 2016 had 'resulted in a significant cut to the supply line of EU workers.'

Dr Andrew Goddard, president of the Royal College of Physicians, questioned how the health service would cope with any more pressure on staffing. 'With research indicating the workforce is at breaking point, anything that impacts the NHS's ability to recruit talented, hardworking professionals is a major risk,' he said. 'We know there are no overnight fixes.'

EU frontline workers were vital to the NHS's ability to keep its services up and running, said Mortimer. 'We can't afford to lose a single colleague from the EU,' he said. 'We are short across the board.'

25 October 2018

www.thebureauinvestigates.com

Key facts

⇨ 303,000 women died due to complications of pregnancy or childbirth in 2015. (page 1)

⇨ In 2016, an estimated one million people died of HIV-related illnesses. (page 1)

⇨ Globally, an estimated 216 million cases of malaria occurred in 2016, compared with 237 million cases in 2010 and 210 million cases in 2013. (page 1)

⇨ An estimated 208 million women of reproductive age who are married or in-union worldwide are still not having their family planning needs met with a modern contraceptive method. (page 2)

⇨ At least half of the world's population do not have full coverage of essential health services. (page 2)

⇨ In 2016, outdoor air pollution in both cities and rural areas caused an estimated 4.2 million deaths worldwide. (page 2)

  • In the same year, indoor and outdoor air pollution caused an estimated seven million deaths, or one in eight deaths globally. (page 2)

⇨ In 2017, 151 million children under five (22%) were stunted (too short for their age), with three-quarters of these children living in the South-East Asia Region or African Region. (page 3)

⇨ WHO estimates that around seven million people die every year from exposure to fine particles in polluted air that penetrate deep into the lungs and cardiovascular system, causing diseases including stroke, heart disease, lung cancer, chronic obstructive pulmonary diseases and respiratory infections, including pneumonia. (page 5)

⇨ More than 90% of air pollution-related deaths occur in low- and middle-income countries, mainly in Asia and Africa, followed by low- and middle-income countries of the Eastern Mediterranean region, Europe and the Americas. (Page 5)

⇨ Around three billion people – more than 40% of the world's population – still do not have access to clean cooking fuels and technologies in their homes, the main source of household air pollution. (Page 6)

⇨ Scientists found that a sleep duration of ten hours is linked with 30 per cent increased risks of early death compared to sleeping for seven hours. (Page 7)

⇨ Study also revealed a 56 per cent increased risk of stroke mortality and a 49 per cent increased risk of cardiovascular mortality for those who slept for more than eight hours. (Page 7)

⇨ Sepsis affects more than 30 million people a year worldwide and kills an estimated 6 million people, of whom nearly 2 million are children. Of those who do survive, 40% will have post-sepsis syndrome, which leaves them with lasting physical and mental symptoms. (page 8)

⇨ Surveys suggest that only 40% of people in Australia have heard of sepsis and only one-third of this group are able to identify a single symptom. Figures are even lower in Brazil where only 14% of the public know what it is. And, although campaigning in the UK and Germany has created an awareness in over 60% of people, knowledge of the warning signs is still limited. (page 8)

⇨ In greater Athens, the number of deaths rises sixfold on heavily polluted days. Mexico City has been declared a hardship post for diplomats because of its unhealthy air. In Bombay, simply breathing is equivalent to smoking half a pack of cigarettes a day. (page 11)

⇨ There were an estimated 10.4 million new cases of active TB in 2016 and 1.7 million people died from the disease, according to the World Health Organization. (page 13)

⇨ HIV continues to be a major global public health issue. In 2017, an estimated 36.9 million people were living with HIV (including 1.8 million children) – with a global HIV prevalence of 0.8% among adults. Around 25% of these same people do not know that they have the virus. (page 17)

⇨ Since the start of the epidemic, an estimated 77.3 million people have become infected with HIV and 35.4 million people have died of AIDS-related illnesses. In 2017, 940,000 people died of AIDS-related illnesses. This number has reduced by more than 51% (1.9 million) since the peak in 2004 and 1.4 million in 2010. (page 17)

⇨ In 2017, 1,792 cases of imported malaria were reported in the UK (1,708 in England, 50 in Scotland, 24 in Wales and 10 in Northern Ireland), 10.8% higher than reported in 2016 (N=1,618) and 15.0% above the mean number of 1,558 cases reported between 2008 and 2017. (page 24)

⇨ In the last ten years (between 2008 and 2017), the total number of malaria cases reported in the UK each year has fluctuated around a mean of 1,558 (95% CI: 1,447–1,668); similar to the mean for the previous ten years (1,533, 95% CI: 1,440–1,627). (page 24)

⇨ Age and sex were known for 1,778/1,792 cases of malaria; of these the majority (67%, 1,188/1,778) were male, consistent with previous years. Males dominated all age groups. The median age was 41 years for males and 40 for females. Children aged less than 18 years accounted for 10% (186) of all cases with known age and sex. (page 24)

⇨ More than 90,000 people in Britain will die over the next three decades unless action is taken to halt the rise in antibiotic-resistant superbug infections. (page 30)

⇨ It is estimated that antibiotics add an average of 20 years to all of our lives. (page 37)

Air pollution

Air pollution can cause both short-term and long-term effects on health and many people are concerned about pollution in the air that they breathe. These people may include people with heart or lung conditions, or other breathing problems, whose health may be affected by air pollution.

Antibiotic resistance

When an antibiotic has been used a lot, it can lose its ability to kill bacteria – the bacteria become 'resistant' to it.

Antimicrobial resistance

A broad term used to refer to 'drug resistance' where a microbe or virus becomes resistant or immune to the drugs used to treat it. Doctors are increasingly concerned that over-prescription of antibiotics has led to some people developing a resistance which means the drugs are less effective.

Communicable diseases

Diseases that you can catch from another person or being. Also known as 'infectious' diseases.

Ebola

An infectious and usually fatal disease that is characterised by severe fever and internal bleeding. It is spread through contact with infected bodily fluids.

Epidemic

Widespread occurrence of an infectious disease.

Food poisoning

Food poisoning is an illness caused by eating contaminated food. It's not usually serious and most people get better within a few days without treatment.

Immunisation

Immunisation is the process whereby a person is made immune or resistant to an infectious disease, typically by the administration of a vaccine.

Malaria

A life-threatening disease caused by a parasite that is transmitted by Anopheles mosquito. With correct medication and precautions, Malaria is preventable and treatable. Only the female Anopheles mosquito can transmit the disease to a human.

Pandemic

A pandemic is an epidemic of disease that has spread across a large region; for instance, multiple continents, or even worldwide

Sepsis

Sepsis is a serious complication of an infection. Without quick treatment, sepsis can lead to multiple organ failure and death.

Smog

Smog is a type of severe air pollution.

Superbug

'Superbug' is a term used to describe strains of bacteria that are resistant to the majority of antibiotics commonly used today.

Tuberculosis (TB)

A bacterial infection spread through inhaling tiny droplets from the coughs or sneezes of an infected person. This is a serious condition but can be cured with proper treatment. Symptoms include a persistent cough, weight loss, night sweats and high temperature.

Vaccine

Vaccines can be prophylactic (example: to prevent or ameliorate the effects of a future infection by a natural or 'wild' pathogen), or therapeutic (e.g. vaccines against cancer are being investigated). The administration of vaccines is called vaccination.

World Health Organization (WHO)

WHO is an agency of the United Nations (UN) that is dedicated to global public health issues.

Zika virus

Zika virus disease is mainly spread by mosquitoes. For most people it's a very mild infection and isn't harmful. But it may be more serious for pregnant women, as there's evidence it causes birth defects – in particular, abnormally small heads (microcephaly). Zika doesn't naturally occur in the UK, however cases in the UK are associated with travel to countries or areas with active Zika virus transmission.

Assignments

Brainstorming

In small groups, discuss what you know about World Health. Consider the following points:

⇨ What World Health issues can you think of?

⇨ What is an epidemic?

⇨ What is smog?

⇨ What is air pollution and what health issues might it cause?

⇨ What is a superbug?

Research

⇨ Choose one of the diseases discussed in this topic and research its history and the development of related treatments. Write a summary of your findings.

⇨ Create a questionnaire to find out how much your class knows about malaria and the ways in which it could be prevented and treated. In which countries is it more prevalent? Write a report which analyses your findings and include a graph to illustrate your information.

⇨ In small groups, choose a country and look at the health issues experienced by its inhabitants. Produce an infogram to show your findings.

⇨ Produce a questionnaire to find out how much sleep your classmates get. Does the amount of time spent sleeping differ between the sexes? Produce a graph to show your findings.

⇨ In pairs, do some research into sepsis. What are the symptoms, causes and treatments of this disease? Do you know anyone who has had sepsis? What was the outcome for them. Write a report on your findings and share with the rest of your class.

Design

⇨ Imagine you work for a health trust that promotes the immunisation of babies and children. Design a poster to highlight your cause.

⇨ In pairs, produce a leaflet about the Zika virus which will be displayed in local hospitals. It should give information about the virus, how it might be treated and information about any travelling restrictions which might apply.

⇨ Choose one of the articles in this book and create an illustration to highlight the key themes/messages of your chosen article.

⇨ Imagine you are working for a charity that is trying to raise awareness of malaria throughout the world. Design a web page that will promote your cause. You can work in pairs or in small groups.

Oral

⇨ As a class, discuss what you think could be done to prevent the spread of malaria throughout the world. How could you inform people of the ways they could protect themselves and their families from this disease.

⇨ In small groups, research Ebola and create a three-minute presentation explaining its causes, and treatment of the disease.

⇨ In pairs, discuss what you have been taught about HIV and AIDS at school. Create a detailed plan for a lesson that will teach pupils of your age-group from developing countries in Africa about these illnesses. Think carefully about what should be included and consider how to make the lesson interesting and relevant to their circumstances.

⇨ As a class, read the article *Brexit risk: more than a quarter of midwives at some London hospitals are EU nationals*. Discuss the impact the referendum has had on staffing levels in our hospitals and the long-term implications of this.

⇨ ## Reading/writing

⇨ Write an article about antibiotic resistance and what is being done to combat this. Write no more than 1,000 words.

⇨ Write a blog post about the use of drones to combat malaria. You should focus on how the drones are used and the efficiency of using them.

⇨ Write a one-paragraph definition of superbugs.

⇨ Read the article *Disease detectives: keeping track of new and emerging infectious diseases* and write a summary for your school newspaper.

⇨ Choose an article and write a one-page summary.

⇨ Write a one-paragraph definition of the word 'Immunisation' and then compare it with a classmate's.

⇨ Imagine you have recently been diagnosed with tuberculosis. Write a blog post expressing your feelings and thoughts. How do you feel right now? What does the future look like? How will your life change?

⇨ The term 'cytokine storm' is mentioned on page 15. Write a short article explaining what this term means.

⇨ Watch the film *Mary and Martha* (2013) and write a review exploring how the director deals with the theme of malaria.

Acknowledgements

The publisher is grateful for permission to reproduce the material in this book. While every care has been taken to trace and acknowledge copyright, the publisher tenders its apology for any accidental infringement or where copyright has proved untraceable. The publisher would be pleased to come to a suitable arrangement in any such case with the rightful owner.

Images

All images courtesy of iStock except pages 7, 10, 13, 14, 16, 18, 19, 31 and 33 Pixabay. Page 29 Morguefile.

Icons

Icons on pages 4, 6, 16, 17, 18, 19 and 21 were made by Freepik from www.flaticon.com.

Illustrations

Don Hatcher: pages 11 & 27. Simon Kneebone: pages 32 & 35. Angelo Madrid: pages 36 & 38.

Additional acknowledgements

With thanks to the Independence team: Shelley Baldry, Tina Brand, Danielle Lobban, Jackie Staines and Jan Sunderland.

Tracy Biram

Cambridge, January 2019